Blueprints
For a Better Body

Steven C. Cummings

Second Edition

Anthem Press, East Derry, New Hampshire

Blueprints for a Better Body

Steven C. Cummings

Published by: **Anthem Press**
Post Office Box 33
East Derry, NH 03041 U.S.A.
anthem-press.com

First Printing 1989
Second Printing 2010, completely revised

Printed in the United States of America

ISBN 0-9677979-7-7

Please Note:

This program contains exercises that, depending on your physical condition, may cause injury. As with any exercise program, consult with your doctor before beginning this routine. If you have any health problems, consulting with a doctor before beginning this program is essential. Use extra care when performing the exercises in this manual, as improper performance could result in injury.

User assumes all risk for performing the exercises described in this course. **Use of this course constitutes a covenant not to bring any lawsuit or action for injury caused by performing exercises illustrated in this course.**
If you do not wish to be bound by this statement, you may return this book to the publisher for a full refund.

Table of Contents

PART THREE: The 8-Week Total Body Makeover

I   Building a Better Body

Your Body Is A Temple

Think of some of the most famous and beautiful cathedrals in the world- St. Marks, the Sistine chapel, or Notre Dame. Early engineers designed these structures not only to stand the test of time, but as remarkable works of art. They are the perfect blend of art and engineering. Form and function. Is the human body any less? From a strictly medical, scientific view, the human body is brilliantly designed. The best engineers in the world could not have built such a strong, adaptable, multi-faceted structure. Each individual organized system -circulatory, nervous, digestive, etc. - serves a definite, pre-determined purpose and is incredibly complex. It takes medical students years just to understand the basic workings of these systems. Combined, these systems can form arguably one of the most beautiful peices of art ever created. The human body is the perfect blend of art and design. Form and function. Just like those famous, wonderfully built cathedrals. If *you* had to build a cathedral, a temple that you had to live in the rest of your life, how would you want to build it? Would you want the doors to sag and squeak and the paint to drip? Would you want it made of thin, weak 2x3 boards with old bricks for a foundation? It's doubtful that anyone would be satisfied to spend their lives in a place like that. Yet many people do just that; Your body truly is a temple, one you must occupy for the rest of your life. Why not make it a strong beautiful one? Anyone can build a better body. It is never too late to make improvements. Start designing your work of art, your temple. Start building a better body now. The blueprints are in your hands.

Acknowledgments

Thanks to my family for always supporting me in whatever I do, no matter how crazy or impractical it might seem at the time...

Part One

Body Design Theory

1 Anatomy & Design

Muscle & fat

The first step in building your new body is learning about the materials you have to work with. When it comes to re-shaping your body, muscle and fat are the two major components. The muscles of the human body are generally divided into three categories:

Smooth muscle

Smooth muscle is found primarily in the walls of hollow organs, such as the intestines. They contract rythmically under the control of the autonomic nervous system.

Cardiac muscle

Cardiac muscle is found exclusively in the heart. Fibers interweave to form a thick, spriral band around the ventricles. Slow, rhytmic contraction is controlled by the autonomic nervous system.

Skeletal muscle

There are over 650 skeletal muscles in the human body comprising up to 45 percent of total body weight. Skeletal muscles are attached to bones, and are what we use everyday for movements of all kind - from weight lifting to chewing food. They are made up of millions of fibers, called *myofibrils*. These myofibrils are arranged in bundles,which form the bulk of a muscle. Although skeletal muscle is considered to be under the control of the voluntary nervous system - because we can consciously decide to move our body - general body movement usually occurs without being consciously aware of it.

(Skeletal)Muscle & fitness

Of the three types of muscle found in the body, skeletal muscle is what needs to be focused on for building a stronger, healthier body. That shouldn't be a problem, since it is the only muslce type under voluntary control. The right program that develops skeletal muscle will develop cardiac muscle as well; As new muscle tissue is added the body must make new vascular capillary networks to feed it. This causes the heart to work harder. It must increase its efficiency, which means it must get stronger. A stronger, more efficient heart is a healthier heart. More and more studies are showing the benefits of skeletal muscle resistance training(such as the program outlined in this book) to reach far beyond just muscular strength.The right resistance training program can develop all of what exercise scientists have identified as the five facets of fitness:

1. Increased muscular size, strength and endurance
2. Enhanced joint flexibility
3. Improved cardio-repiratory efficiency
4. Increased body leaness
5. Reduced risk of musculoskeletal as well as cardio-vascular injury. This last benefit is a result of the first four.

Although traditiional aerobic training such as running and bicycling can be very beneficial, focusing primarily on resistance training of the skeletal muscles will achieve a greater level of fitness in the most efficient manner.

What makes a muscle?

Skeletal muscles can be huge, such as the gluteus maximus, or buttocks, or tiny, such as the strapedius of the middle ear. As mentionied previously, muscle consists of bundles of cylindrical fibers that contract, or shorten with chemical or electrical stimulation, creating a pulling force. These muscle fibers are generally divided into two types: white, "fast twitch" fibers which are activated during quick, high intensity activity such as weight trainingand red "slow twitch" fibers which are activated during long, low intensity exercise such as running or bicycling.

Developing muscle

Developing muscle is really a process of damage and repair. Exercising overloads muscle fibers, causing microscopic damage. This signals the body to release chemicals that begin the process of replicatng muscle cells, which ultimately creates thicker, stronger fibers. The body does this to prepare the muscle to cope with the increased workload. Rest and recuperation is often under-emphasized or completely ignored in exercise programs, but it is during rest that the real development of muscle and fitness takes place.

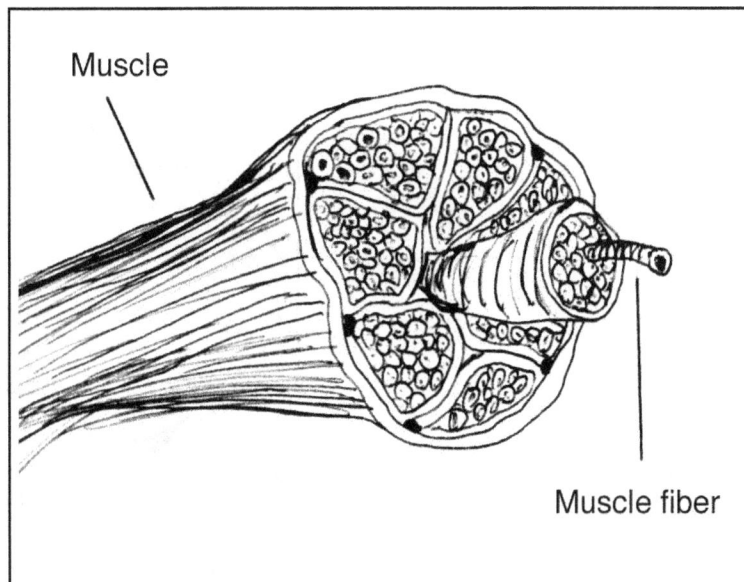

A Muscle consists of millions of fibers like these. Developing a muscle is a process of damaging the microscopic muscle cells in these fibers, and allowing them to be repaired.

Body fat

Most everyone is very familiar with body fat and most everyone would like to have less of it. Body fat, or *adipose tissue*, is located not only under the skin, but also around kidneys and eyeballs, in bones and breasts and within the abdomen. Its major purpose is for reserve food fuel, but also acts as an insulator against heat loss, and supports and protects internal organs. We all have a predetermined number of fat cells in our body which can only be changed by surgical removal, as in a liposuction procedure. Fat cells will expand or shrink depending on body needs, and those who are very lean may still have a large number of fat cells.

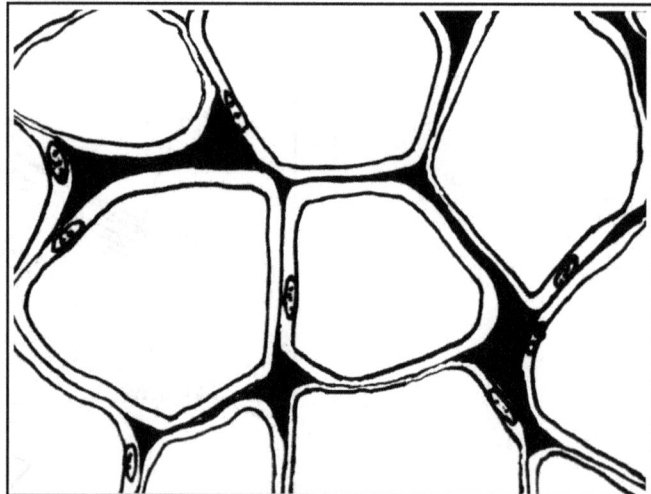

Human Fat Cells(Adipose tissue) under the skin.

A person's body leanness is measured by percentage of body weight. For example, if a man weighs 170 pounds and 17 pounds of that is fat, he would be said to have10 percent body fat. The body fat percentage for the average male is 16 percent, while the average female has 26 percent body fat. The ideal for men is generally agreed to be 10 to 12 percent and the ideal for women is between 16 and 18 percent. To see real definition in the abdominal area, usually a bodyfat percentage of 10 or less is required of both sexes. Although some bodyfat is required for overall good health, it is not unusual for top bodybuilders and fitness athletes to have just 2 or 3 percent body fat. This is probably the lowest level of body fat that can be achieved without risking health.

Designing your body

The first step in designing your new body is deciding what areas you want to improve. Do you want to lose fat around your waistline? Build a bigger chest? Sculpt and define your legs? The anatomy diagrams on the next pages can help you to identify areas that need improvement. Some of your other goals may not be immediately visible, such as lower blood pressure, increased cardiovascular health or more overall enegry. While this program can help you achieve all of these goals and more, having a definite focus of what you want to achieve is an essential first step. The next step is breaking those goals down into small, easy to reach steps; if you want to increase your chest size, focus on adding more weight or more repetitions on the bench press. If you want to lower your blood pressure, pay attention to the sodium in your diet. Take all of your health and fitness goals and write them down. Doing so will make them more real and give you a stronger focus.

Areas to
focus on

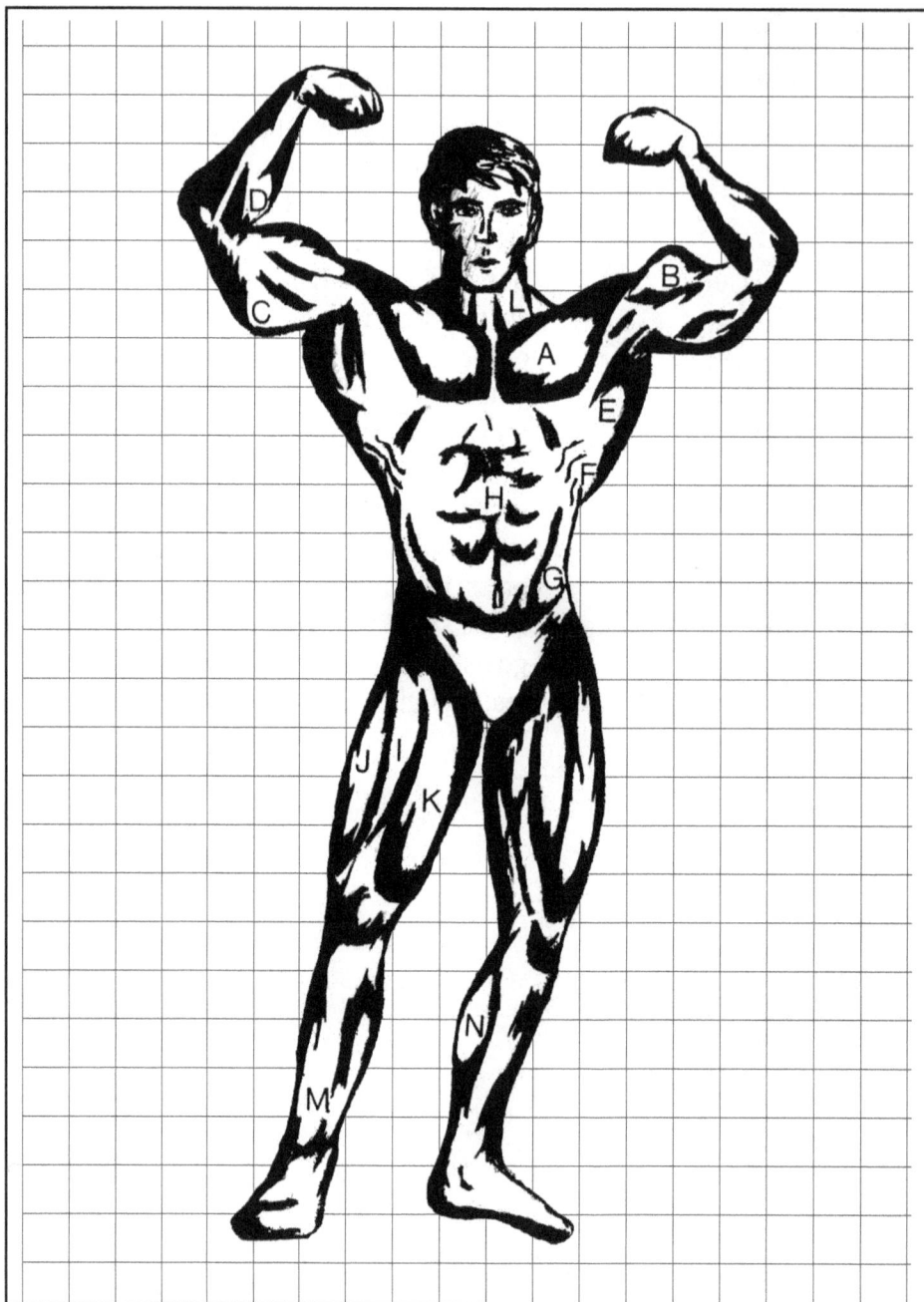

Front View

A. Pectoralis Major("Pecs")
B. Biceps
C. Triceps
D. Flexor Carpi Radialis
E. Latissimus Dorsi("Lats")
F. Serratus Magnus
G. Obliques Externus Abdominis

H. Rectus Abdominus("Abs")
I. Quadriceps Femoris("Quads")
J. Vastus Lateralis
K. Vastus Medialis
L. Sternocleido-Mastoid
M. Tibialis Anticus
N. Gastrocnemius

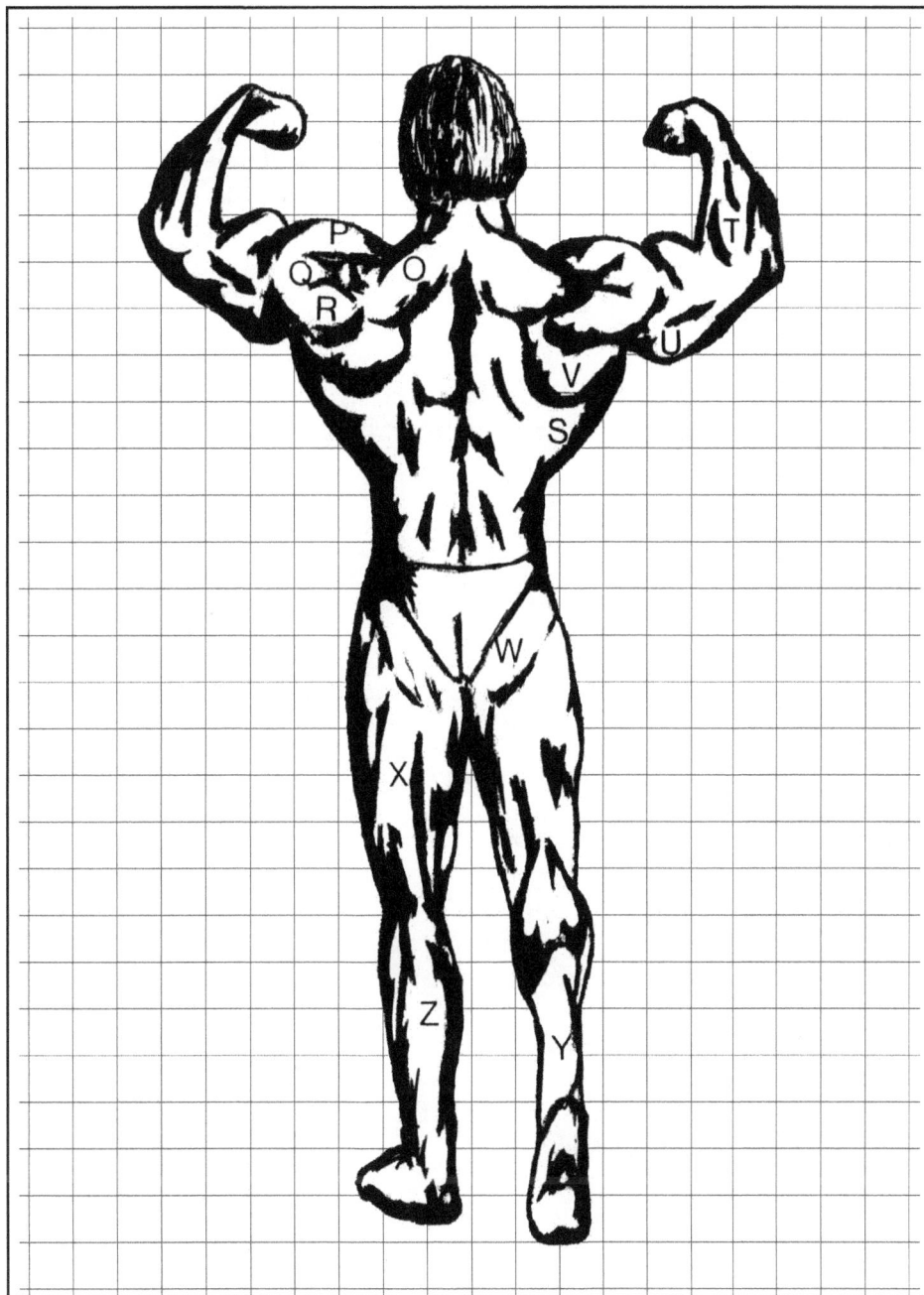

Rear View

O. Trapezius("Traps")	U. Triceps
P. Anterior Deltoid	V. Teres Major
Q. Medial Deltoid	W. Gluteus Maximus("Glutes")
R. Posterior Deltoid	X. Biceps Femoris
S. Latissimus Dorsi("Lats")	Y. Soleus
T. Extensor Carpi Radialis	Z. Gastrocnemius("calves")

2 Basic Body Construction Principles

Study these basic principles for training carefully. The better you understand and apply them, the more effective your training will be:

Intensity

In order to stimulate maximum muscle growth you must exercise with the highest intensity possible. For years the trend was(and still is)long, low intensity, multiple set, high volume weight training. While this type of training might work for those genetically gifted weight trainers, or those using steroids, for the genetically average(like most of us), results are mediocre, at best. Evidence has mounted over the years proving that brief, high intensity training produces better results than traditional resistance training programs. There are several factors that determine intensity:

Momentary muscular failure

After selecting the appropriate weight on an exercise, you should perform as many repetitions as possible. When you can no longer complete a repetition in good form, despite your greatest effort, you have reached momentary muscular failure. It is absolutely essential to carry each exercise to the point of failure. If each set is not carried to this point, very little muscle growth will occur.

Number of sets

Many resistance trainers believe that multiple sets of the same exercise will build more muscle. In most cases, this is not true. One set of each exercise, brought to the point of momentary muscular failure is all that is needed to stimulate growth.

Arthur Jones, the inventor of Nautilus machines , used to compare exercise to flipping on a light switch. You only need to flip the switch once to get the bulb to light. Flipping it again and again would do no good except to waste time. Similarly, when you work muscle fibers to the point of failure, you only need to do it once to set the rebuilding process in motion. A second set will work the same set of fibers over again, which would only serve to extend your recovery time.

Volume of work

Ten to twelve exercises per workout should be plenty enough if performed in the correct manner. Short, high intensity workouts build muscular size and strength. Long, low intensity workouts build muscular endurance.

Time between exercises

Do not rest too long between exercises - never more than a minute. Try to gradually reduce the time between exercises every workout, until there is almost no rest between them at all. Doing this will increase the overall intensity of the workout.

Neurological Efficiency

Neurological efficiency refers to a person's ability to recruit muscle fibers; electrical impulses from the nervous system determine what type and how much of each muscle fiber type is activated during exercise. All muscle fibers are never fully activated; a percentage of fiber is always left in reserve. Some can activate more than others, however. Those who have a high neurological efficiency can recruit more overall muscle fibers.

Repetitions

The right number of repetitions for an exercise varies from individual to individual, based on that persons dominant muscle fiber type. Those with predominantly "fast twitch" fibers are generally stronger but can perform only a small number of repetitions. Those with predominantly "slow twitch" fibers may not be able to handle as much weight, but can perfrom many more repetitions. About 80% of the population has mixed fiber types, meaning they have a roughly equal amount of "fast twitch" and "slow twitch" fibers. It has been determined that, for most resistance trainers,(those with mixed fiber types), the ideal number of repetions for a given exercise is between 8 and 12. At this point you may be asking, "How do I know what *my* dominant fiber type is? There is a simple but effective way to test your neurological efficiency to determine he ideal number of repetitions for your training. It will be covered in the "preliminaries"section of this book.

Tried&true

In the 1940's and 1950's, weight trainers were using some very simple and very effective methods to really pack on muscle mass. This was well before the development of steroids, and yet these trainers were able to build some incredible physiques. Many of these training techniques were forgotten. Some have slowly been making their way back into the gym. Presented here are some of these old, but very effective methods;

Breathing squats

Squats are one of the most difficult and uncomfortable exercises to perform. They are also one of the most productive in terms of muscle growth. Squats place enormous intensity on the hips, thighs and buttocks. These areas are the strongest and largest muscle groups on the body. Exercising these groups intensly will cause muscle growth all over the body, possibly due to the release of growth hormone that is believed to occur after placing great stress on the hip joints. Weight trainers in the old days used to really pile on the weight adding five or ten pounds every workout and taking one or two full, deep breaths between reps, hence, the name "breathing squats". They would always try to complete twenty repetitions, which is why they were sometimes also referred to as "twenty-rep squats". At the end of just one set of heavy breathing squats, most trainers were completely out of breath and panting. Breathing squats are a powerful method to add muscle mass fast, all over the body. While they are far from easy to perform, the results are well worth the effort.

Rib cage expansion

Performed right after a set of heavy breathing squats, straight arm pullovers with a dumbell can actually increase the size of your ribcage. Many people find this surprising, but it was common practice in the gyms of the 1950's. In photos of bodybuilders and weight trainers from 40 or 50 years ago, the enlarged ribcage is easy to identify. An expanded ribcage can make a chest and back appear wider, larger and thicker. This adds a unique look of power that has sadly fell out of fashion.

Expanding the shoulder girth

Would you like to have wider shoulders? For women, this usually isn't a primary goal, but for men wide shoulders is a symbol of strength and power. Building the muscles of the shoulder can certainly help, but expanding your shoulder girth can really make a dramatic difference in attaining powerful, wide shoulders. Weight trainers of the old days used to perform extra wide-grip chin-ups, claiming it actually increased

Concentrate on multiple-joint

Big, multiple joint movements such as barbell bench press, overhead press, behind the neck press, deadlift and rows used to be the cornerstone of a workout in the gyms of the 1950's. Unfortunately, most gym-goers today concentrate on isolated movements that are found on many modern day weight machines. Pec deck flyes, shoulders raise, bicep and tricep curls have their place and can be useful, but concentrating on "big" movements involving multiple joints and larger muscle groups will produce much better overall results.

Other considerations

There are some other training principles and considerations that you may or may not be aware of, but which are vitally important for your training success:

Exercise order

Generally, your largest muscles should be exercised first, working down to the smallest muscles, but when specializing on a specific muscle group, that goup should have priority and be exercised first. All of this has been taken into account, and your workouts prepared accordingly in the eight week total body workout described later in this book.

Frequency of workouts

On this program, you should rest at least 48 hours between

workouts. Adopting a Monday, Wednesday, Friday schedule would be the most effective, with Wednesday reserved exclusively for aerobic/endurance development. Exercising three times a week will provide all the necessary stimulation for muscle growth, and allow enough time for recovery. With high intensity training, two or three workouts per week is all that is needed for maximum effect.

Progression

In order to gain muscle mass you must attempt to increase your workload each workout. You can do this by increasing the amount of resistance or the nuber of repetitions or both. For example; if your repetitions guidline were 7 - 9 for the biceps curl, you would choose a resistance that would allow you to perform 7 repetitions in good form. When you are able to perform 10 repetitions with the same weight, you should increase the resistance at your next workout by 5% and attempt to perform 7 repetitions.

Aerobic exercise

In general, there are two kinds of exercise, *aerobic* and *anaerobic*. Anaerobic exercise is brief, high intensity exercise, such as resistance training. It involves mostly "fast twitch" muscle fibers which use glycogen stores in muscle cells as the primary source of fuel. Long, low intensity activity, such as jogging or swimming, is aerobic. It involves mostly "slow twitch" muscle fibers which use oxygen as the primary source of fuel. For the most part, anaerobic exercise (parcticularly weight training), is the most effective and effi-cient method for developing overall fitness. As described in chapter one, building muscle mass leads to positive gains in all five facets of fitness. However, aerobic exerise can and should still play an important part in your fitness program. Besides improving the condition of the heart and lungs, aerobic exercise can also improve the appearance of your muscles by developing the slow-twitch fibers that are involved when performing any aerobic activity. In order to derive the benefits of aerobic activity, your heart rate must be elevated and sustained for at least 10 minutes, three times per week. The correct heart rate for aerobic conditioning is 70% to 85% of your *maximum heart rate*. A simple formula used to determine maximum heart rate is to subtract your age from 220. For example, a 35 year olds maximum heart rate would be 185. He would then need to get his heart rate elevated to at least 130(70%) but

not more than 157(85%) to get any aerobic benefits.
Follow the chart below to determine your target heart rate
range for aerobic conditioning:

Age	Maximum HR	Target HR	10 sec. pulse count
20	200	140-175	23-29
25	195	137-166	23-28
30	190	133-162	22-27
35	185	130-157	22-26
40	180	126-153	21-25
45	175	123-149	21-24
50	170	119-145	20-24
55	165	116-140	19-23
60	160	112-136	19-22
65	155	109-132	18-22
70	150	105-128	18-21
75	145	102-123	17-21
80	140	98-119	16-20
85	135	95-115	16-19

The most convenient way to make sure you are reaching and
sustaining your target heart rate is with an eletronic heart rate
monitor. These can be purchased at most sporting goods
stores at a relatively low price. If you are a member of a
gym, most cardio equipment has a built in heart rate monitor,
and these are usually very accurate. If youcan't afford or
don't have access to a heart rate monitor, you can still
monitor your heart rate by periodically taking a 10-second
count of your pulse. Refer to the heart rate chart for
10-second pulse counts for the targetheart rate for your age.

Breathing

Many people recommend certain ways to breathe while exercising, but as long as you don't hold your breath, there really is no "correct" way to breathe. With the exception of the " breathing squats" and pullovers, which require you to breath deeply, there really are no rules. Some people prefer to breathe out during the concentric or lifting portion of the exercise, others concentrate on breathing in a deep, rhytmic pattern. Whatever is comfortable and works for you is fine. When in doubt, just breathe naturally.

Keeping record

Keeping accurate records is essential to determine your progress in this program. The workout sheets provided have spaces for record keeping for your convenience. Simply fill in the date, weight and repetitions with each workout. It is also a good idea to periodically weigh yourself and make a written record of it.

Rest and recuperation

Rest is perhaps the most overlooked area of concern in exercise, yet it is only during rest that muscle repair and growth occurs. When the body is stressed, it requires more rest to recuperate. High-intensity exercise is very stressful on the body, and allowing adequate time to rest afterward is essential for progress. If you find that you have stopped making progress with your training, try adding an extra day of rest between workouts. Contrary to popular belief, the stronger and more advanced you become, the *less* work you need to do. When you find yourself reaching plateaus, cut back in workouts per week, or cut back in number of exercises. This is often the easiest way to break a sticking point or plateau in your training. If you have been training intensely for months or years without a break, you may have to take a whole week or two off to fully recover.

N-T-F (Not To Failure) Workouts

Although in general, all exercises should be taken to the point of muscular failure, there are times when a lower-intensity workout might be beneficial; in cases of temporary minor injury or illness, or on days when you feel particularly tired and weak, for whatever reason. Under such circumstances, a N-T-F workout might be an appropriate consideration.

Safety issues

It is important to be vigilant about training safely; injuries are quite common among resistance trainers. Almost all of these injuries can be avoided if some basic rules of safety are adhered to;

Warming up

It is always a good idea to warm up before doing any heavy, intense exercise. Just fifteen to twenty minutes on a treadmill or stationary bike can warm up muscle and joints enough to prevent most injuries, therefore, performing 20 minutes of aerobic activity(sustaining your target HR)before your resitance training would be an excellent way to accomplish two goals at once.

Stretching

As an additional safeguard against injury, it is a good idea to stretch before and after exercising. It is really a very simple and quick procedure that should not be avoided. Not only does it prevent injury, but it will help you to maintain and possibly increase your flexibility as well. The recomended movements include: Head rotations, pectoral stretch, hamstring stretch, quadriceps stretch, lat stretch, groin stretch, side twists and the hanging stretch. All of these movements are illustrated in part two of this book, and should only take thirty seconds each to perform.

Proper form

When performing each repetition, special care should be taken to control the movement at all times throughout the range of motion. Never throw or jerk the weight. Count 2 or 3 seconds during the positive, or lifting portion of a repetition, and count 4 or 5 seconds on the negative, or lowering portion.

Protecting your joints

Keep in mind that resistance training will place stress on the joints. Ultimately, resistance training will improve the condition of joints by building up the muscle, tendon and ligaments in and around them, but care must always be taken; Never "lock out" joints during resistance training, and be careful of movements that have the potential to hyper-extend a joint, such as machine biceps curl or pec deck flyes. Protecting your joints now will mean a relatively pain free future.

Training partners

When engaging in any high intensity resistance training program, it is always a good idea to train with someone who can "spot" you in case you run into trouble. This is especially true if you are using free weights and are training to failure. Not only are they there for your safety, but also to make sure you do not " cheat" on any exercises by shortening the range of motion or using improper form, and to provide encouragement as well.

Muscle soreness

If you are a beginner at resistance training you can expect some muscle soreness after your first workout. Muscle soreness is usually caused by a build up of lactic acid, and can occur as soon as 12 hours after your workout and may last as long as 3 days. In any case, all workouts should be avoided until most of the soreness has dissappeared. If the degree of soreness has not lessened or improved within three days, your may have an injury and should consult your doctor.

Special techniques

There are many special techniques that can increase intensity, and therefore results. Most of these techniques should be reserved for intermediate to advanced trainers, but some can be safely used for all serious resistance trainers. Some of the best specialized techniques are explained here;

Pre-exhaustion

When an isolation exercise for a certain muscle group is immediately followed by a multiple-joint movement for the same muscle group, it is known as pre-exhaustion. Let's say, as an example, that you completed a set of Nautilus biceps curls. Bringing it to a point of momentary muscular failure, you would have exhausted your biceps muscles.

If you were to then immediately perform a set of chin-ups, this would bring your biceps to a further degree of exhaustion. The Nautilus biceps curl is an isolation movement used to pre-exhaust the biceps. Immediately performing a other multiple-joint exercise such as the chin-up allows muscles such as the latissimus dorsi and pectorals to bring the biceps muscles to a point beyond momentary muscular failure. Performing the isolation exercise and the multiplejoint movement with less than three seconds between them is absolutely essential for the best results. Some the exercises in the last five weeks of the eight week total body make-over have been arranged in a pre-exhaustion format.

Negatives

When a weight is raised, the movement is called the *concentric,* or positive contraction. When the weight is low ered, the movement is called the eccentric, or negative contraction. Contrary to popular belief, the negative portion of the exercise is the most important and the most productive in terms of muscle growth. Most people can handle about 40% more weight on a negative repetion than they can on a positive one, and that's one reason why muscle growth is so dramatic; handling more weight requires a muscle to grow stronger, and a stronger muscle is a bigger muscle. Although negatives can be productive, they are also inherently dangerous because of the heavier weights that are required. Most negative movements would require several assistants to perform, but some can be done by yourself. Some of the simpler negative movements have been incorporated into this training program.

Partial reps

Upon reaching a point of momentary muscular failure, it is possible to create an even greater degree of tension by performing quarter or half movement with the same weight.

Forced reps

After reaching a point where it is impossible to perform even partial reps, your training partner can assist you in per forming a few more repetitions. By helping you to lift the weight, he is actually reducing the resistance, allowing you to perform a few full repetitions. Doing this will bring you to a point beyond momentary muscular failure, causing greater muscle tension and greater muscle growth.

Progressive negative tension

Progressive negative tension is just what it sounds like; a gradual increase in the amount of tension during the negative contraction. This is accomplished by increasing the amount of time it takes to lower the weight with each repetition. With every exercise performed, the weight should be lifted in 2 to 3 seconds, lowered in 4,, lifted in 3, lowered in 5, lifted in 3, lowered in 6, and so on until you reach momentary muscular failure. If your tested ideal repetitions guide turns out to be more than 12-14 reps for any exercise, do not increase the time lowering the weight past 10 seconds. For example; when you reach your 7th positive repetition, you would lower the weight in 10 seconds, and on your 8th repetiton you would lower it for 10 seconds again and continue lowering it for 10 seconds until mometary muscular failure. If your repetitions guide were more the 12-14 reps and you did not follow this 10 second rule, your workout could take hours, and remember, we are trying to keep the workouts as brief as possible in order to keep the intensity level high. You can try progressive negative tension on some of your favorite exercises - or all of your exercises if you want. Some of the benefits of P.N.T. training are; improved concentration, improved exercise form and increased exercise intensity.

3 Equipment & Devices

Free weights & machines

Machines or free weights?
It has been a subject of popular debate for many years, ever since the introduction of the first Nautilus machine in the early 1970's. Since then, there has been an explosion of muscle building and fitness devices on the market, from ab rollers to electro-muscle stimulators, all guaranteeing a shortcut to health and fitness. While some of this equipment is useful and productive, others are clearly not worth the cost.

Free weights

With the invention of the plate loading adjustable barbell in 1902, resistance training finally became measurable and progressive. Adjustable dumbells, barbells and weight benches are still very popular today and are collectively known as "free weights". They are inexpensive and readily available at most department or sporting goods stores. Most major gyms have a free weight area as well. They are usually favored among "hardcore" bodybuilders, some who still believe they are somehow more effective than machines, such as Nautilus. While free weights are inexpensive and very productive if used correctly, they are also inherently dangerous; Lifting heavy barbells above your head, chest or behind your back leaves much opportunity for injury. Extra care should always be taken when using free weights. Having a training partner would also be a wise choice to prevent injury.

Machines

Weight machines, particularly Nautilus machines, are in many ways superior to free weights; they are much safer, since you cannot "drop" a weight on you or become trapped under a weight you cannot handle, the best ones offer rotary resistance, which applies equal force throughout the range of motion and can greatly enhance results and the resistance can be changed quickly and easily with just the movement of a metal "pin". If you have access to them, you are better off focusing most of your training on Nautilus or some of the other machines available to you in the gym, and supplementing just a few free weight movements. If not, free weights will certainly work.

Bodyweight equipment

Some equipment uses primarily your own bodyweight as resistance, although, technically, you will have to strap free weight onto you to make any progress using this equipment. Despite their obvious limitations, some of this equipment, if used properly, can produce some startling results;

Parallel dip bars

Parallel Dip Bars have their origins in the world of gymnastics, where gymnasts train on two long, parallel wooden bars. In the early days of bodybuilding and fitness, the bars were built much shorter and stronger, and eventually evolved into a strong, compact unit with strength training in mind instead of gymnastics. Most major gyms have at least one "dipping station" now, either as a free standing unit or part of a larger peice of equipment. Some are even designed to offer variable assistance by providing lift at your feet, helping you to lift your bodyweight if you are unable to do so on your own. It is not

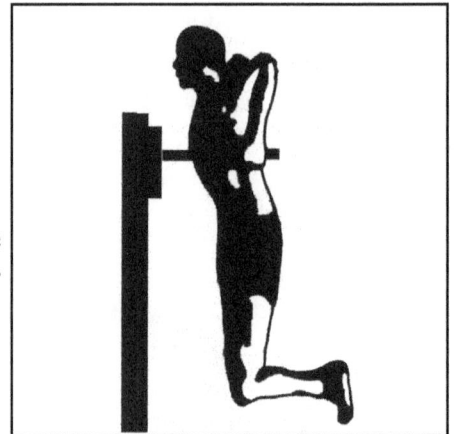

uncommon for some trainers to develop their strength on this exercise to the point where they strap 50, 75 or 100 pounds around their waist. In the early days of fitness, the parallel dip was known to develop such a powerful upper body that some called it the "upper-body squat". Some have even suggested that a powerful body could be built with just squats and parallel dips alone.

Chin up bar

Like the Parallel Dip Bars, this peice of equipment is most effective when weight is added progressively to a special belt strapped around the waste. Most gyms have some type of chin bar, but if you don't have access to one, they can be purchased at a very low cost at most department or sporting goods stores, and installed in any solid doorway. Chin-ups are an excellent multiple joint movement for developing the upper body, and this device is one not to overook.

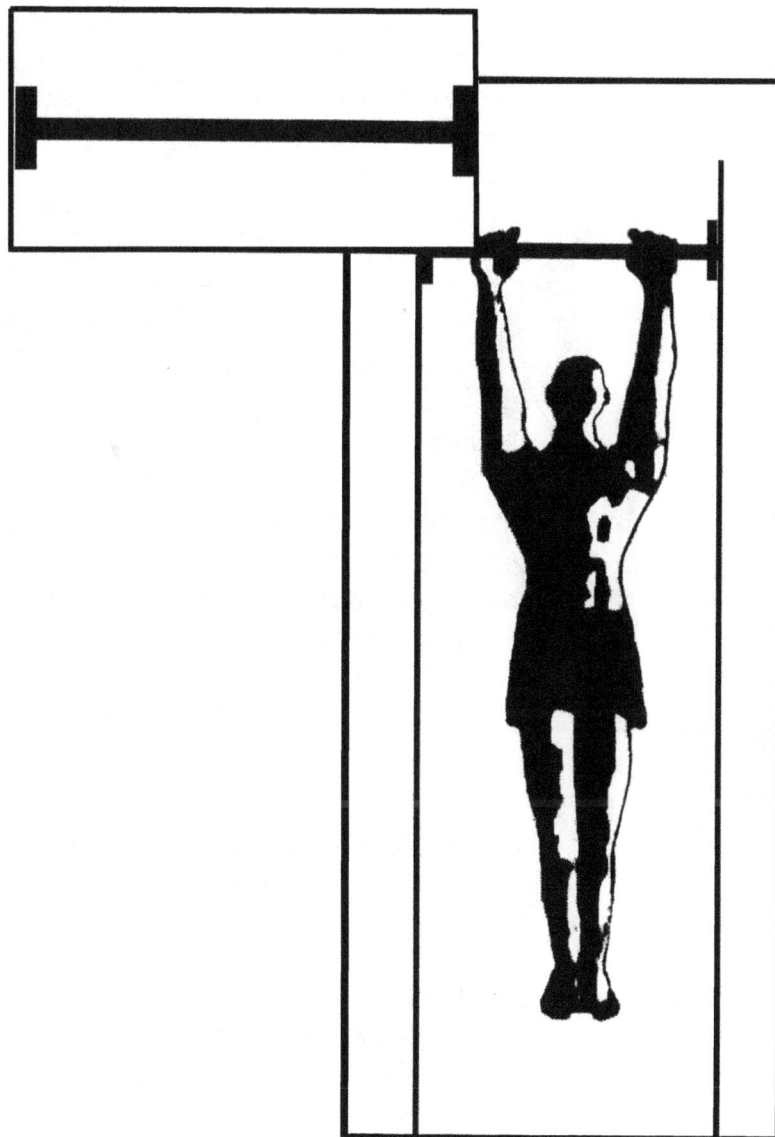

Weighted dip belt

If you want to develop your body quickly, these belts are essential equipment. Dipping belts are simple in design. They are basically a regular weight lifting style belt with a strong metal chain hanging in the front. They are designed to hang loosely from the hip structure while allowing free weight plates to suspend between the legs by the chain. They are usually built out of very strong material, and can handle quite a bit of weight. Dipping belts are not very easy to find, but they are well worth the effort.

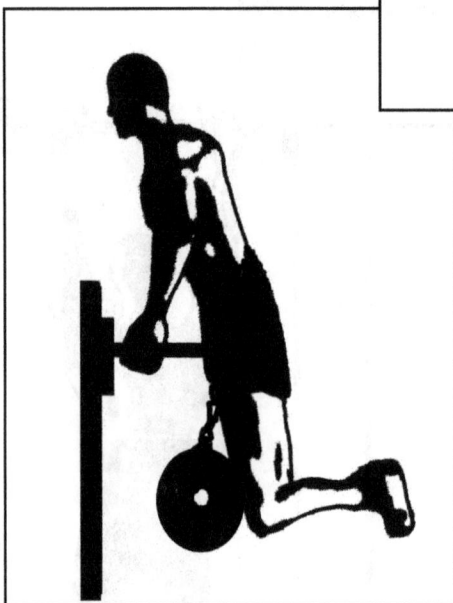

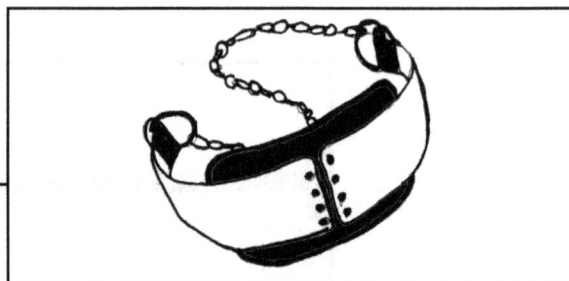

Aerobic equipment

Most gyms have such a large selection of aerobic or "cardio" equipment that it is sometimes hard to decide which one is best to use. As long as the peice of equipment provides a heart rate monitor, the best choice is one that you feel most comfortable with:

Treadmill

The old standby, the treadmill, is still a very good, very effective aerobic conditioning tool. The best ones have hand grips that measure your heart rate and displays it on a screen in front of you.For most people, a brisk walking pace is all that is necessary to bring the heart rate up to target range.

Stair steppers

As it's name implies, stair steppers are based on the natural action of climbing stairs. The best ones are automated, with variable resistance and pre-programmed starting levels. When using stairsteppers, be sure to carefully monitor your heart rate, as it is easy to exceed the high end of your target HR range.

Elliptical machines

Elliptical machines are relatively new on the fitness scene, havinggained popularity only in the last ten years or so. They are set up like a combination of the treadmill and the stair stepper, only your feet are guided through the range of motion in a smooth, elliptical arc. The major advantage of these machines is the greatly reduced stress on knee and ankle joints as opposed to the treadmill and stairstepper. If knee and ankle joint discomfort are an issue for you, the elliptical machine might be a better choice.

Trampoline

Not too long ago, trampolines were all the rage, but, as fads often do, they lost their popularity quickly. If you have a trampoline or can pick one up cheaply, they can provide an adequate aerobic workout if used properly. The advantages are a reduced impact on joints and, obviously, they are a lot more fun than other aerobic equipment. They are inherently dangerous, however, and many accidents have occured as a result of them, so use with caution, and always remember - watch that heart rate!

Stationary bikes

A good stationary bike can provide an excellent aerobic workout while reducing pressure and impact on the knee and ankle joints. The best ones electronically monitor not only heart rate but time, speed, distance and calories burned. Some even offer a variety of resistance levels to challenge you as become stronger and develop more aerobic endurance.

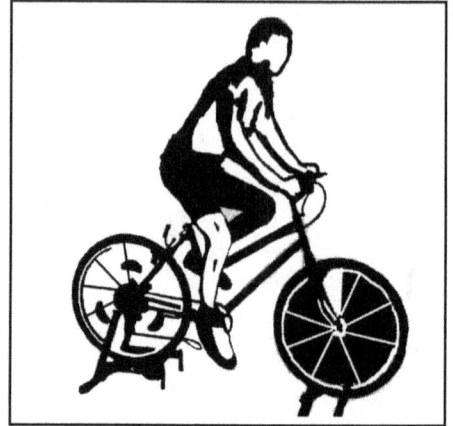

Swimming pools

Although a swimming pool may not technically be a "device" or peice of "equipment", swimming is such a great form of aerobic exercise it cannot go without mention here. If you have access to a pool, or even a lake or the ocean, consider adding a good 15 to 20 minutes of swimming to your routine once in a while. Swimming is considered one of the best "low impact" exercises available, and will help you avoid wear and tear on your joints. The only drawback is that you must use the 10-second pulse rate check to monitor your heart rate.

Jump rope

A simple peice of rope, used properly, can be an excellent aerobic conditioning tool. Jumping rope as a form of exercise used to be quite popular years ago, but has since fallen by the wayside as new, more technical cardio machines have become increasingly popular and easy to use. It can still be an effective and fun device in your aerobic conditioning program. Remember to check your pulse or wear a heart rate monitor, however.

Snow shoes

For those of you who live in snow country, a pair of snow shoes can make an excellent investment. Modern day snowshoes are nothing like the big, bulky contraptions of the past; these newly designed shoes are small, lightweight and easy to use. As always, monitor your heart rate, for a novel aerobic workout.

Cross country skis

Like snow shoeing, cross country skiing can be a great way to enjoy those dark winter months and get an effective aerobic workout at the same time. If you have never been cross country skiing before, it will take some time just to develop the coordination necessary for the movements. If you prefer, you can also use one of the older cross country ski machines, like Nordic trak. Both will provide a good, low impact aerobic workout.

Other devices

Abdominal devices

Over the last few years, several abdominal training devices have flooded the market. Torso track, ab roller, ab rocker - they all promise the same result; a lean, strong waistline. Do any of these really work? Sure. They all work. But you can get the same results from simple abdominal exercises (as outlined in this book) and a floor mat. Also, most gyms have very good abdominal machines available that will work just as well, if not better than those infomercial ab contraptions.

Medicine balls

Medicine balls used to be quite common in gyms across the country in the 1940's and 1950's. Today they have become something of an antique, and difficult to find. If you can locate one, they can be very useful in building explosive strength and developing upper body muscle mass. They operate on the principles of *plyometrics*, which is a method of training that exploits the natural, in-born muscle protective mechanism known as the *myotatic reflex*. Plyometric training can produce some incredible muscle mass quickly, but the potential for injury is very high.

Electro-muscle stimulators

Electo-muscle stimulators consist of machines that deliver a small electrical charge to a muscle, causing it to contract, much in the same manner as when exercised. The value of these devices is limited, as they simply contract a muscle without adding progressive resistance. They can be useful, however, as a supplement to your regular resistance training routine; Muscle stimulators have been shown in some studies to improve muscle recovery after a workout, and reduce muscle soreness, possibly by stimulating blood flow and reducing lactic acid build-up that occurs after anaerobic exercise.

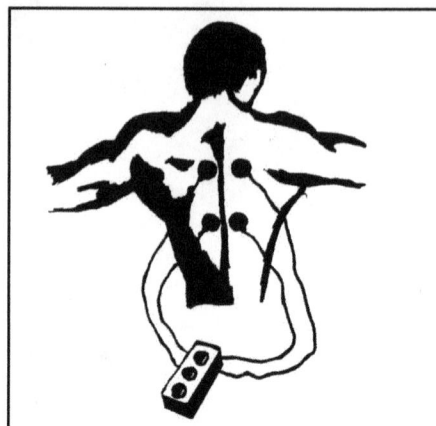

4 Using Your Mind for Fitness

Mind over muscle

We've all heard of mind-over-matter, and scientists have known for a long time that there is some degree of truth to the idea; In drug testing, a certain percentage of patients always respond just as well to a sugar pill as to the real drug when they are not aware of it being so. This "placebo effect" is established fact in the scientific community, and is an interesting example of the power of the mind to affect the body. It is not necessary for you to "trick" yourself, however, to tap into this power. There are several techniques that can help you use your mind to improve your results from this training program:

Visualization

Visualization has been used successfully for years to improve sports performance, motor skills of all kinds and even medical conditions. Stories of terminally ill cancer patients using visualization to help improve their conditions, and in some cases even shrinking tumors completely, are not uncommon. Put simply, visualization is making pictures in your head. They can be in the form of a movie or a still picture, color or black and white. You can add sound, taste and smell, as well as heat, cold or pressure to the pictures, if desired. The main point is to choose your goal - decide what you want - and to see yourself as already having it, making it as realistic as possible. Here is an example of how a visualization session for this program might work:

1) Sit or lie down in a comfortable position.

2) Relax your body; Start with the muscles of your face and work down. Breathe in through your nose and tighten the muscles of your face. Hold for 3 seconds. Then relax while breathing out through the mouth. Now move on to the neck, shoulders, chest, etc., all the way down to your feet.

3) Visualize the muscles in your body(refer to anatomy diagram if necessary), See and feel them growing, getting stonger. Now form an image of any extra fat deposits. See the fat just metling away, shrinking until you can see the sculptured muscle underneath. Try to feel what it is like to have a strong, lean, flexible body, with chiseled abs, well developed shoulders and arms, and a powerful, defined chest. See yourself walking, tall and proud and strong. Feel what it is like to walk with confidence in your new head-turning physique.

This might seem ridiculous to some people, but visualizing like this before each training session will improve your results tremendously. Arnold Shwartzenegger was well known to use visualization during his bodybuilding days, and has often credited it with his success. You can do it as often as you like,but try for at least once a day. The process above is just an example; You can be as creative as you like. Just remember to focus on your goals. Some people find that focusing on a picture of a bodybuilder or fitness personality with a body that they would like to have can be very helpful with the visualization process. At the very least, visualization will give you a motivational boost, and besides, like daydreaming, it can be a lot of fun.

Self hypnosis

Most psychologists believe in the unconscious mind, but have made very little progress in understanding exactly what it is and what it does. There a lots of theories, but very little solid facts. One thing is certain; the unconscious mind is capable of some very unusual and powerful things, if it can be reached. One way to reach it is by hypnosis. Psychologists are not sure exactly how it works, but most agree that is does indeed work, and many use it regularly in their practice. There are some truly amazing stories involving hypnosis; stories about people controlling asthma and pain and dissolving warts right before your eyes. Stories of people "losing" their diabetes while in trance state and even changing their eye color. It is possible to hypnotize yourself, as well. Thefollowing is a simple exercise in self-hypnosis that you can use to enhance your results:

1) Sit or lie down in a comfortable place. Do not cross your hands or legs, just let them rest at your sides.

2) Relax your body using progressive relaxation. (Follow the directions in Visualization, step 2).

3) Focus on the words "I am getting lean and strong". Repeat them slowly and clearly in your head. Clear your mind of everything else. When stray thoughts enter your mind, just gently push them away and return to the phrase "I am getting lean and strong". Continue this for 10 to 15 minutes. You can set an alarm if you have trouble gauging the time.

Like visualization, this technique will work best before your workout or before going to sleep.

Lucid dreaming

Lucid dreaming is the state of being consciously aware that you are dreaming while you are actually dreaming. It is a state of being conscious and awake while remaining fully asleep. What that basically means is that you can control the outcome, content and nearly every aspect of your dreams. When you learn the proper techniques, it's like having Alladin's lamp in your head, better than any virtual reality machine you could imagine. Every wish you ever had can come true at night while you lay safely in bed sleeping. The potential of lucid dreaming is far greater than simple wish fulfillment, however. Dream control opens up a whole world of possibilities and potentials. One such possibility is the ability to physically affect the body through dreams. In fact, Dr. Stephen LaBerge of the Stanford University Sleep Research Center has been studying lucid dreaming for years and has discovered that certain physical movements and manipulations performed deliberately during lucid dreams can have a very real, tangible effect on the physical body. So, let's get down to what this means to you: You can build any body you want in your dreams. Once you learn the techniques of dream control you can make your muslces grow and be as lean as you like. You can weight train in your dreams as well; you can lift thousands of pounds if you want. What effect this will have in the real world cannot be predicted. The simplest technique to induce lucid dreams is state testing. The procedure for state testing is as follows:

1) Begin testing your state of consciousness by asking yourself "Am I dreaming?" or "Is this a dream?" throughou the day.

2) After asking the question, begin to check your environment for inconsistencies; read a passage in a book or newspaper,then re-read the passage. If it changes in any way, you are dreaming. Check to see if you can fly; jump up and see how long you can stay up there. If you remain in the air for even a second or two longer than seems normal, you are dreaming.

3) If you discover that you are not dreaming, try to imagine what it would be like if you were; imagine where the inconsistencies would be and what they would be like; how the words would be changed, what it would be like to be flying. Try to imagine this as vividly as possible.

State testing works by sheer probability; If you test your state enough times, eventually you will find yourself in the dreamstate. Leaning how to lucid dream does require some effort, but once learned could have some startling results in terms of growth, and will enrich your life in many other ways as well.

NLP

NLP stands for Neuro-linguistic programming. It was developed in the mid 1970's by an information scientist, Richard Bandler, and a linguistics expert, John Grinder. It is an unusual, controversial science dealing with how the brain processes and codes information. NLP therapists have been known to cure life-long phobias in a half-hour, help children and adults overcome "learning disabilities" in less than an hour and even eliminate allergic responses in only a few sessions. Some NLP techniques can be very useful in enhancing your growth results. the following is one such example:

1) Think of the time during puberty when you began to grow taller, bigger. A time when new muscles began to appear all over your body. If it is an image, notice where it is placed in your personal space; is it up and to your left or right out in front of you? Is it a movie or a still picture? Notice where and how the memories are displayed.

2) Begin to think of your exercise and weight training routines as "like" puberty. Make an image of yourself exercising and getting stronger, your muscles growing larger and fat melting away. This image must be displayed in exactly the same way as your memories of puberty - same colors, distance and style (movie or still picture).

3) Now take these images of you exercise and growing and place them in the same personal space as your memories of puberty.

This technique may seem overly simple, but what you are doing is actually very powerful; you are re-encoding your brain to respond to this exercise routine in a similar manner as it did to puberty. Performing this technique once or twice should be all that is needed.

Meditation

Meditation is an ancient practice, dating back thousands of years. There are many different forms and techniques, but some of the best involve progressive relaxation of the body and controlled, focused breathing. In many ways, it is similar to both self-hypnosis and visualization, with the addition of the breathing patterns. The following meditation technique can be helpful for finding and relaxing tension in the muscles of the body:

1) Relax your body using the progressive relaxation method (see visualization, step 2).

2) Begin breathing in a four-step method; breathe in through the nose for a count of four and hold for a count of three. Breathe out through the mouth for a count of four and hold for a count of three. Try to concentrate the breathing in the stomach (diaphragm), rather than up in the chest.

3) Bring your attention to the muscles of the neck. Notice any tightness or tension in them. Imagine drawing your breath into the muscles. As you exhale, release any tension and relax. Now bring your attention to the back muscles. Draw your breath "into" the them, releasing all tension as you exhale. Remember to count as you breathe.

4) Continue for ten to fifteen minutes, scanning your body for any tension, and releasing it as you exhale.

Prayer

Prayer is also an ancient practice, dating as far back as mankind itself. Every major religion in the world practices prayer in one form or another. Appealing to God, Jesus or simply the Universe for your health and fitness - can be helpful and healthy on many levels. Whether or not you believe in a higher power, prayer has been shown in several controlled studies to have positive affects on health and should be considered an effective means of improvement. Some might cringe at the thought of praying for a fit body, but as I said in the Introduction of this book,, your body truly is a temple. Asking God for help with building a strong, healthy body is not selfish or vain, it is a way of showing respect; to yourself and - if you are a believer - to the higher power that created you.

Use the following prayer as a guideline; substituting names or phrases where necessary to suit your particular tastes and beliefs:

God, I ask you to grant me a strong, healthy, fit body. Help me to choose healthy foods to eat, so that I might fuel my body with the right nutrients. Help me to stay focused and disciplined in my workouts, so that I might become a stronger, healthier person. Help my heart and lungs to become stronger, my joints to become more flexible and resistant to injury. Help me to become lean, shedding unecessary body fat, and help my muscles to grow larger and stronger. Help me to achieve this that I might respect myself and the body you have given me more. Amen.

The brain-spinal column connection

The spinal cord (a) descends from a lower section of the brain called the medulla oblongata (b). Branching out from the cord along the length of the spine are 31 pairs of nerves, some for each section of the spine - cervical, thoracic, lumbar and sacral. The spinal cord itself only travels two-thirds of the way down the spinal canal, leaving 9 pairs of nerves at the bottom which must travel a long distance before spraying out the bottom to form what is known as the cauda equina (c). Each spinal nerve (d) consists of bundles of long fibers of individual nerve cells. Some of these fibers carry signals from the skin and muscles to the spinal cord, while others carry information from the spinal cord to glands and muscles. These fibers send and receive information from all parts of your body. Ultimately, the signals are processed in the brain (e). There is a powerful connection between the brain and spine and therefore it is readily and easily accessed and influenced by our thoughts. Something to keep in mind when practicing some of the techniques covered in this chapter.

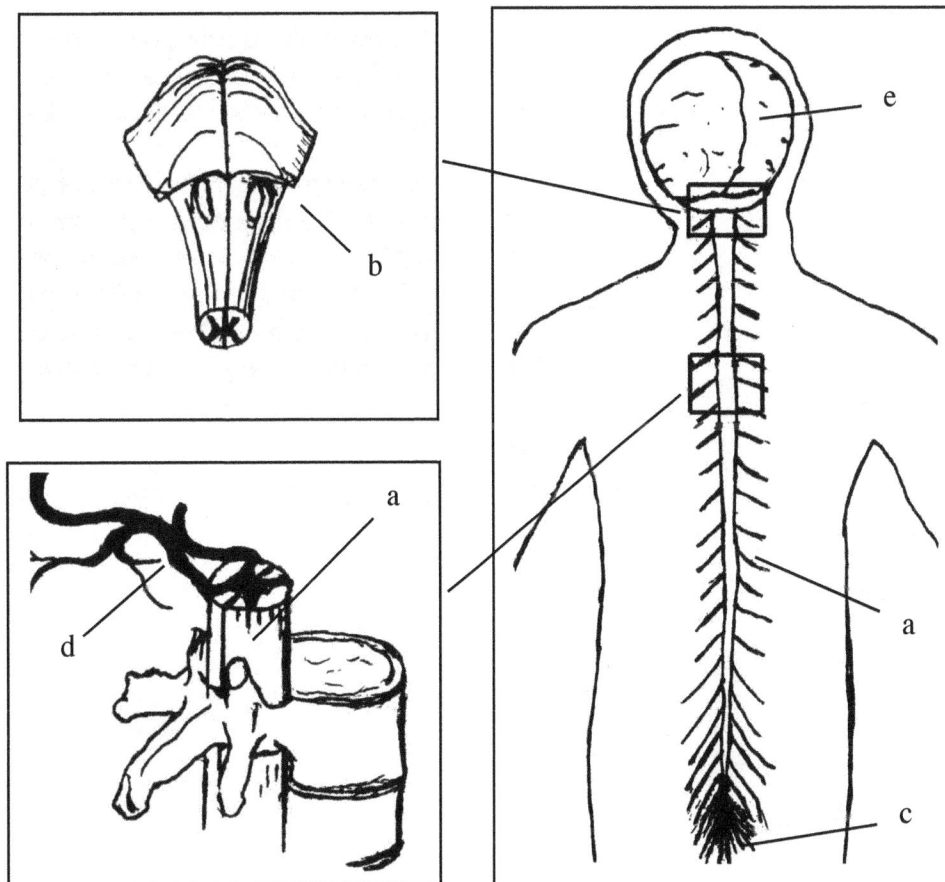

5 Nutrition

Designing a diet

Designing the perfect diet for maximum muscle building, fat loss and fitness can be confusing and frustrating. There are so many new "diet" plans out there - all promising fantastic fat loss and good health - that it is hard to decide which one is right for you. The best "diet" is really no diet at all, but a permanent change in eating habits based on some of the most basic nutritional standards, and some new findings about the way our bodies use food;

The basics

With all the new dieting and nutritional information available today, it is sometimes easy to forget the basics. There are several things our bodies need to function properly and maintain health:

Charbohydrates

Carbohydrates are sugars and starches and are the main energy sources of metabolism. A diet rich in carbohydrates will provide fuel for exercise. Despite what the latest low-carb diet program might be suggesting, carbohydrates are essential for good health, and will not make you fat if you are careful to eat the right foods (more on this later). Whole grain breads, pasta, fruits and vegetables are the best sources for carbohydrates and should make up 50-60% of the diet.

Proteins

Proteins are needed for growth and repair of tissues and cells. Each protein contains hundreds of amino acid units. There are twenty specicfic amino acids, eight of which must be obtained from a balanced diet. The remaining twelve can be made by the body. The need for protein is slightly increased when the body is under stress, as it is when intensely exercised. Some good sources of protein include; lean meat, fish, tofu, eggs, dry beans and nuts(including peanut butter). Protein should make up between 15% and 25% or your diet. Keep in mind that the body can only absorb 20-30 grams of protein in one sitting.

Fats

Fats are a structural component of cells and, like carbohydrates, provide energy for metabolism. Many people think of fats in a negative way, but actually it is essential to have some fat in the diet to maintain good health. There are three kinds of fats; saturated, monosaturated, and polyunsaturated. Of these, saturated fat is the one to be avoided. It increases cholesterol and the risk of heart disease. Saturated fats are found mostly in meat and dairy products, while mono-unsaturated and polyunsaturated fats can be found in olive oil, avocados, fish and vegetable oils. In recent years there has been much attention to the health benefits of omega-3 fatty acids. It has been shown to improve brain function, protect the heart and reduce joint inflammation. Good sources of omega-3 fatty acids include; fatty ocean fish such as herring, salmon, and tuna, black currant oil, flaxseed oil, borage seed oil and green vegetables. Total fats in your diet should be between 15% and 25%.

Vitamins

Vitamins are regulators of metabolism and ensure the healthy functioning of the brain, skin, nerves, muscles and bones. Some vitamins enable energy to be released from food. Multi-vitamin supplements should be considered for any balanced diet, but use with caution; any vitamin can be dangerous if taken in excess. Multi-vitamins with no more than 100% RDA are best.

Minerals

Minerals are an essential part of any diet and a balanced eating plan provides most people with plenty enough to meet the recommended daily allowances. Two important minerals in health are sodium and potassium. They are both important factors in blood pressure regulation, muscular contraction and fluid balance. The typical American diet is far too high in sodium and very low in potassium. Some good sources of potassium include; bannanas, green leafy vegetables and most vegetable juices.

Fiber

Although it passes through the digestive tract unchangeed, fiber is an essential part of a balanced diet. High fiber diets have been shown to decrease the risk of certain types of cancer and to help keep the digestive tract healthy and functioning well, preventing constipation and other disorders. It can also help you with your fat loss goals by providing a feeling of fullness so you want to eat less, and by breaking down into acids that help the fat burning process. Try to eat at least 30 grams of fiber per day, a little with each meal.

Water

Water determines the volume of blood in our circulation and is essential for metabolism. About 60% of the human body is composed of water. You should try to drink one 8-ounce glass of water every 2 hours while you are awake. Making that water ice cold can help your efforts to become lean; your body will burn extra calories to heat the water up to your body temperature.

Calories

Calories are a measure of energy from the proteins, fats and carbohydrates that we eat. While counting calories for every meal is tedious and unecessary, it can be helpful to evaluate your current caloric needs when deciding how much to eat. One way to determine how many calories you need to support your current bodyweight is to write down everything that you eat over the next three days, add total calories and then divide by three. Use that number as a general guide to how many servings of food to eat per day (refer to calorie/serving guide, figure A, later in this chapter) If one of your primary goals is losing excess fat, then consider reducing total servings, (thereby reducing calories). Even if you decide to continue to eat the same number of servings, you can still reduce bodyfat if you concentrate on building muscle through high intensity weight training. Changing nothing else will still produce results. Just one extra pound of muscle requires over 3,000 calories per month to support. If you gain just 5 pounds of muscle (which is a very realisitc goal), you will require over 15,000 calories per month to support it. Fat will disappear because the calories that used to support it will now be used to support muscle mass - which is usually much more attractive!

What is a serving?

A serving, whether it is a protein, vegetable or grain, should be about the size of a deck of cards, or about the amount that could fit in the palm of your hand. This equals about 20-25 grams. If in liquid form think 6-8 oz.

How often should I eat it?

It is better to spread your servings out over the day in five or six small meals , than in three big ones. Eating every two or three hours will help keep blood sugar levels stable. Avoid getting hungry, as hunger can trigger a starvation response, encouraging storage of body fat.

The food pyramid

The USDA's *old* food pyramid is a good system for basic nutrition. Use it as a *general* guide to good dietary habits:

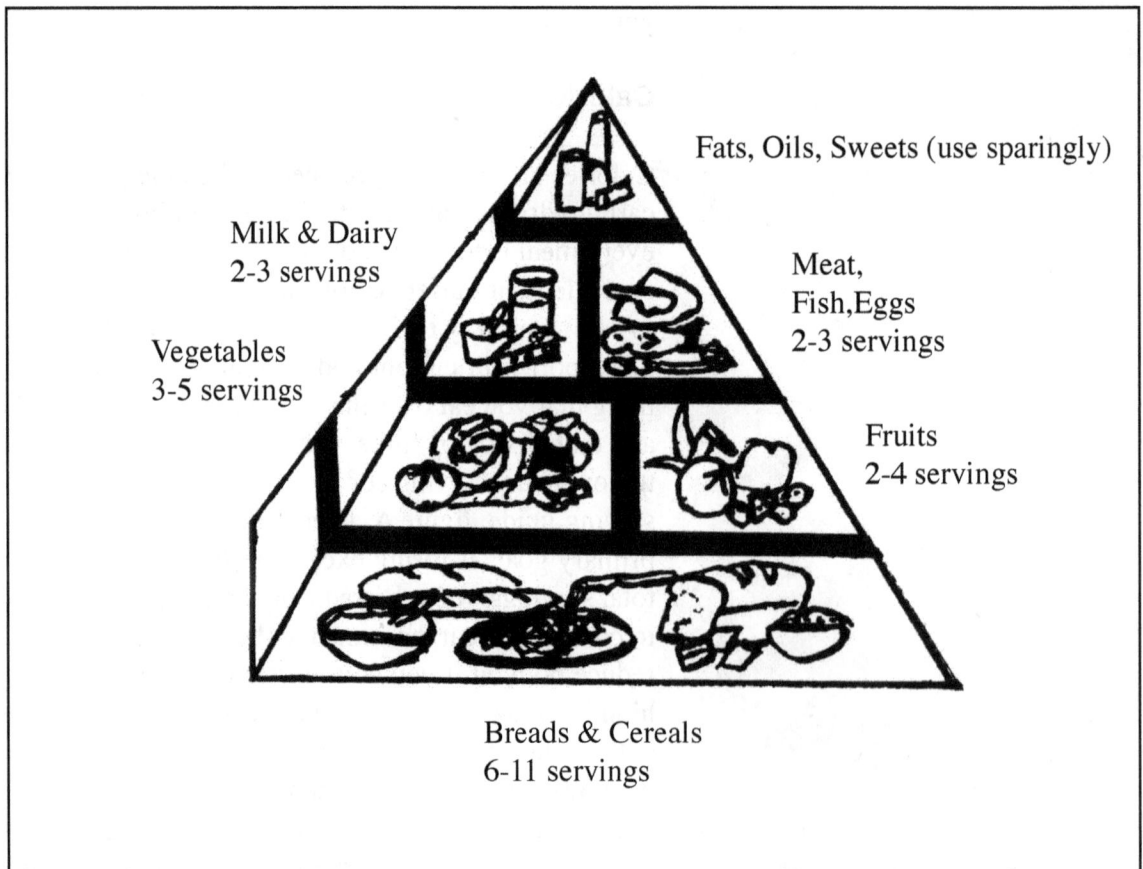

Fats, Oils, Sweets (use sparingly)

Milk & Dairy
2-3 servings

Meat,
Fish,Eggs
2-3 servings

Vegetables
3-5 servings

Fruits
2-4 servings

Breads & Cereals
6-11 servings

Calorie/Serving Guide - Figure A

1800 Calories

Lean protein:	3 Servings
Dairy:	2 Servings
Fruit:	2 Servings
Vegetable:	3 Servings
Bread/Cereals:	6 Servings
Fats/Oils:	1 Serving

1900 Calories

Lean protein:	3.25 Servings
Dairy:	2.25 Servings
Fruit:	2.25 Servings
Vegetable:	3.25 Servings
Bread/Cereals:	6.25 Servings
Fats/Oils:	1.25 Serving

2000 Calories

Lean protein:	3.5 Servings
Dairy:	2.5 Servings
Fruit:	2.5 Servings
Vegetable:	3.5 Servings
Breads/Cereals:	6.5 Servings
Fats/Oils:	1.5 Serving

2100 Calories

Lean protein:	3.75 Servings
Dairy:	2.75 Servings
Fruit:	2.75 Servings
Vegetable:	3.75 Servings
Bread/Cereal:	6.75 Servings
Fats/Oils:	1.75 Servings

2200 Calories

Lean protein:	4 Servings
Dairy:	3 Servings
Fruit:	3 Servings
Vegetable:	4 Servings
Bread/Cereal:	7 Servings
Fats/Oils	2 Servings

2300 Calories

Lean protein:	4.25 Servings
Dairy:	3.25 Servings
Fruit:	3.25 Servings
Vegetable:	4.25 Servings
Bread/Cereal	7.25 Servings
Fats/Oils	2.25 Servings

2400 Calories

Lean protein:	4.5 Servings
Dairy:	3.5 Servings
Fruit:	3.5 Servings
Vegetable:	4.5 Servings
Bread/Cereal:	7.5 Servings
Fats/Oils:	2.5 Servings

2500 Calories

Lean protein:	4.75 Servings
Dairy:	3.75 Servings
Fruit:	3.75 Servings
Vegetable:	4.75 Servings
Bread/Cereal:	7.75 Servings
Fats/Oils:	2.75 Servings

2600 Calories

Lean protein:	5 Servings
Dairy:	4 Servings
Fruit:	4 Servings
Vegetable:	5 Servnings
Bread/Cereal:	8 Servings
Fats/Oils:	3 Servings

2700 Calories

Lean protein:	5.25 Servings
Dairy:	4.25 Servings
Fruit:	4.25 Servings
Vegetable:	5.25 Servnings
Bread/Cereal:	8.25 Servings
Fats/Oils:	3.25 Servings

2800 Calories

Lean protein:	5.5 Servings
Dairy:	4.5 Servings
Fruit:	4.5 Servings
Vegetable:	5.5 Servnings
Bread/Cereal:	8.5 Servings
Fats/Oils:	3.5 Servings

2900 Calories

Lean protein:	5.75 Servings
Dairy:	4.75 Servings
Fruit:	4.75 Servings
Vegetable:	5.75 Servnings
Bread/Cereal:	8.75 Servings
Fats/Oils:	3.75 Servings

The glycemic index

The glycemic index (GI) is a measure of how much and how quickly foods affect our blood sugar levels. They are generally rated on a scale of 0 to 100. The higher the number, the higher the GI of that food, and the greatest spike in blood sugar levels. Sharp fluctuations in blood sugar can cause a number of health problems, and high GI foods have been linked to obesity, diabetes and other metabolic diseases. Learning to eat a diet of primarily low GI foods can go a long way in helping you to lose fat, build muscle and improve health in many areas. In fact, research recently published in *The Lancet* suggests that a high GI diet leads to an increase in body fat, loss of muscle mass and early signs of diabetes, while a low GI diet can reverse these effects.

The truth about low-carb diets

With the increasing popularity of low-carb diets, many people have come to believe that carbohydrates are the enemy. This is simply not true. Eating an abundance of fruits, vegetables, whole grains and even pasta is the cornerstone of a healthy diet. It's the *type* of carbs you eat that makes the difference. The key is to focus on unprocessed, unrefined carbohydrates, such as stone-ground whole wheat bread, fresh fruits and vegetables, nuts and legumes. These usually have a low GI rating (refer to the list of low GI foods on the next page). Highly refined carbohydrates like cereals with added sweeteners, white breads and juices with high fructose corn syrup have high GI ratings and are the real enemy of your health and fitness goals. Low carb diets may help you lose weight in the short run, but will its high saturated fat, low vitamin and mineral foods be good for your health in the long run?
Hundreds of studies have proven that a carbohydrate rich, low GI diet is a healthy way to shed fat and build muscle.

Using the glycemic index to your advantage

Whenever possible, you should choose low GI foods for your meals. You don't necessarily have to eat ONLY low GI foods, but eating a low GI food with every meal will make a tremendous difference in overall health and fitness. The following is a list of some common foods with low GI values:

Lean Proteins	Vegetables	Fruits	Breads & Grains
Chicken breast	Artichoke	Apples	Brown rice
Lean ground beef	Broccoli	Apricot	Whole rice
Ham	Cauliflower	Avocado	Wild rice
Trimmed pork	Celery	Berries(any)	Barley
Game birds	Cilantro	Cantaloupes	Whole oats
Fish(any kind)	Eggplant	Cucumber	Whole wheat
Eggs	Green beans	Grapes	Pasta(all kinds)
Cottage cheese	Mushrooms	Melon	Buckwheat
Tofu	Peas	Kiwi	Bulger
Protein powders	Spinach	Mango	Corn(canned)
Crab	Squash	Orange	Muesli
Shellfish	Sweet Potato	Nectarines	
Clams	Onions	Peaches	
Skim milk	Okra	Pears	
	Yam	Plums	
		Strawberries	

Using high GI foods to your advantage

Beleive it or not, some high GI foods can be very useful for your body sculpting goals;

The 30- minute "window"

Recent research suggests that the most important repair and rebuilding work takes place in the first 30 minutes after intense weight training exercise. This is a "window" of opportunity to supply the right materials to assure that the muscle is repaired optimally. Exercise scientists have found that combining a high GI value drink with protein and consuming it within the first 30 minutes after a workout can enhance exercise recovery tremendously. Mixing a protein powder supplement containing 15-30 grams of good quality protien with a high GI drink like Gatorade would provide an excellent post-workout recovery drink, and should be considered a necessity after your workouts.

High GI foods and the immune system

Just as there is a window of opportunity to enhance growth results, there is also a window of opportunity of a more detrimental kind; Intense exercise can temporarily suppress immune function, leaving you open to viruses, bacteria and infection. Research has shown that intense exercise depletes glycogen stores, causing blood sugar levels to drop and the body to release the stress hormone cortisol, which temporarily impairs the immune system. It appears this affect can be lessened, if not entirely avoided by simply drinking a high-GI beverage like Gatorade *during* your work out. Several double-blind, placebo controlled studies have shown that consuming high-GI carbohydrates during exercise boosts immune system function by preventing dips in blood sugar.

Other Considerations

The "cheat" day

One thing to consider when designing your diet, is to allow yourself one day per week to eat anything you want; pizza, ice cream, chocolate chip cookies -anything.   Many exercise and nutrition programs recommend this "cheat" day, and for good reason; it offers tremendous motivation and mental support to stick to a healthy diet. The thought of never being able to eat their favorite foods again often compels many people to never even attempt a healthier eating plan. Knowing that one day each week you can have that chocolate cake can make a huge difference, and if you eat healthy the rest of the week, your body won't even notice.

Nutritional supplements

There is a lot of hype in the sport and nutritional supplement industry, and very little that actually works as it is claimed to. Sifting out the hype from the fact, what works from what is useless can be a daunting task, but usually, if you wait long enough,the ones that really work will rise to the top. The following supplements have at least some research behind them to support the claims. Although a resistance training program like the one in this book will produce great results by simply following a healthy, balanced eating plan, some of these supplements can enhance your results tremendously:

Creatine monohydrate

Creatine has quickly become the most popular sports supplement in history, primarily because it delivers some very big results. Dozens of clinical trials have proven it is effective in adding muscle bulk, and possibly strength. The major side effect is gastrointestinal distress, which occurs during the initial, high-dose "loading" stage. Also, since creatine can affect the kidneys, those with kidney disorders should avoid it.

HMB

HMB is short for beta-hydroxy beta-methylbutyrate. It is a metabolite of the essential amino acid leucine. HMB is involved in the synthesis of muscle tissue, and studies show that supplementing with HMB can increase lean muscle mass by several pounds and improve recovery after intense exercise.

L-Arginine

This amino acid has been shown to increase lean body mass in several studies. This is especially true when combined with HMB. L-arginine seems to increase protein synthesis, and supplements have been used to speed wound healing, improve the immune system and treat certain cardiovascular conditions.

L-tyrosine

L-tyrosine is an amino acid found in most foods. In high doses - 1,500 to 3,000 mg - it has been shown to improve focus and concentration, which is helpful in high intensity training, and also to actually improve strength within 1/2 hour. This sounds farfetched at first, but L-tyrosine has been shown to increase neurotransmitters in the brain, particularly norepinephrine. This suggests that the mechanism behind the sudden strength increase is due to the nervous system recruiting more muscle fibers. More muscle fiber recruitment means you can lift heavier weights, and heavier weights equal bigger, stronger muscles.

L-theanine

L-theanine is another amino acid, found in large amounts in green tea. In several studies it has been shown to stimulate several neurotransmitters in the brain, leading to a state of calm and relaxation. It has also been shown to block the release of cortisol, the hormone released after instense exercise or stress that can limit muslce growth and impair the immune system. Taking 100 to 200 mg. of L-theanine 30 minutes before and again immediately after your workout can be very helpful for muscle recovery.

Methoxyisoflavone

Methoxyisoflavone is a compound resulting from a European pharmaceutical company's search for a drug that would reverse muscle wasting in hospitalized patients. Methoxyisoflavone worked, causing patients to gain several pounds of lean muscle mass, but the pharmaceutical company lacked the resources to get it approved in the United States. There are several methoxyisoflavone supplements on the market now, some combining protein and other substances in the same product.

Myostatin blockers

Myostatin is a genetic protein found in the human body that limits how big a muscle can grow. Myostatin blockers are relatively new supplements that use a natural compound derived from a rare marine algae called *cystoseira canariensis* that binds to and neutralizes myostatin. In theory, blocking myostatin can lead to incredible muscle gains. Few controlled studies have been performed on these substances yet, but the results of those few studies are promising, and supplementing with myostatin blockers might be worthwhile to consider.

Phosphatidylserine

Like L-theanine, Phosphatidylserine is a substance that essentially blocks cortisol, the stress hormone released through intense exercise that can limit muscle growth, slow recovery time and impair the immune system. Supplementing 400 to 1,200 mg of Phosphatidylserine 30 minutes before your workout can make a huge difference not only in muscle growth results, but in maintaing health.

Protein powders

A good, quality protein powder is the cornerstone of any sound nutritional supplement regimen. Whey protein is considered one of the best, but there are many other types including; milk and egg proteins, rice proteins and various combination products. A good protein product can make snacks quick , convenient and healthy. Look for ones with low fat-to-protein ratios, and 15-30 grams of protein per serving.

ZMA

ZMA is a combination of zinc monomethionine, magnesium aspartate and vitamin B6. The combination of these compounds can increase free testosterone(which can help build more muscle mass), reduce muscle fatigue by minimizing lactic acid build-up in muscle tissue, and significantly decrease cortisol levels. These supplements appear to work best when taken at night, before bed.

Part Two

Body Design Practice

6   The Exercises

Aerobic exercise

Aerobic exercise should always be performed *first,* before any of the stretching or weight training exercises. Doing so ensures that your muscles will be thoroughly warmed up, more receptive to stretching, and less likely to be injured during resistance training. Be sure to keep your heart rate up to target range for 15-20 minutes. Refer to chapter 2 for more information on aerobic conditioning.

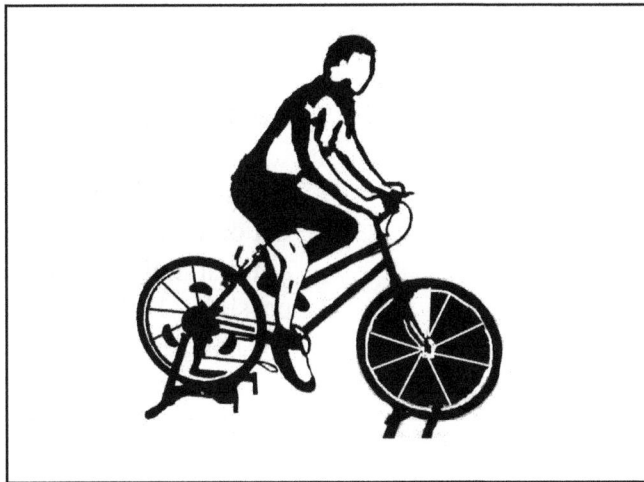

Perform some type of aerobics first, for 15-30 minutes.

Stretching

After 15-20 minutes of aerobic training, you should spend a few minutes stretching. Not only can this help to increase flexibility and prevent injury, but it can also improve your results from weight training by encouraging more muscle fiber recruitment. On the following page are some simple, basic stretches, and should only take, in total, 5 minutes to perform:

Head rotations

Bend your head dow so that your chin touches your chest.
Rotate your head carefully, slowly in a circular motion.
Continue for 15 seconds.

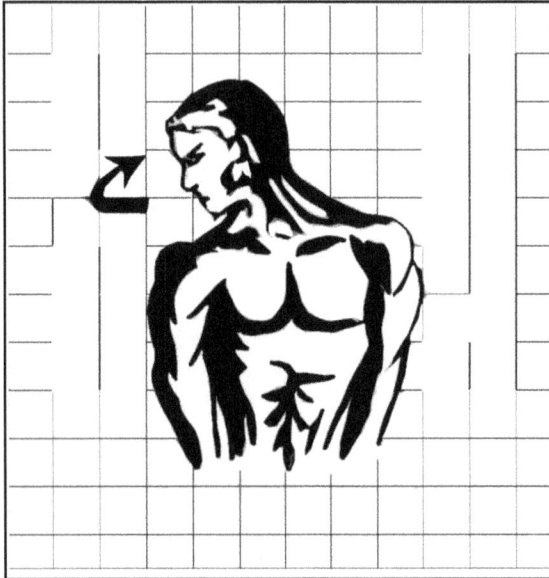

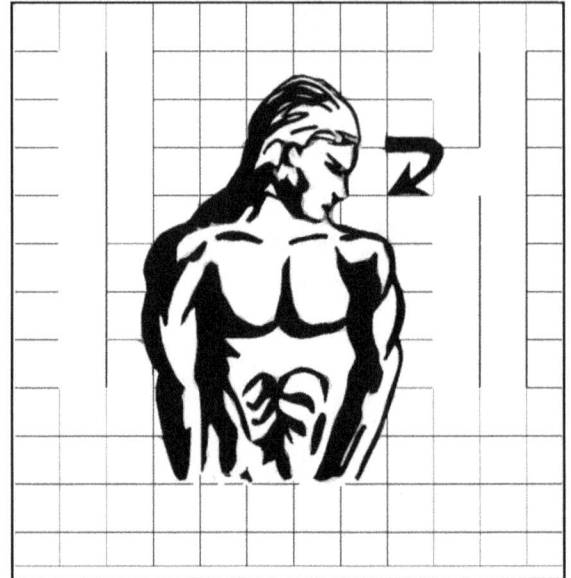

Pectoral stretch

In a standing position, face a wall and place your right hand
flat on it, keeping your fingers pointed to the right. With your
arm parallel to the floor, twist your torso to the left as far as
possible. Hold for 15 to 30 seconds. Repeat procedure using
left hand and arm.

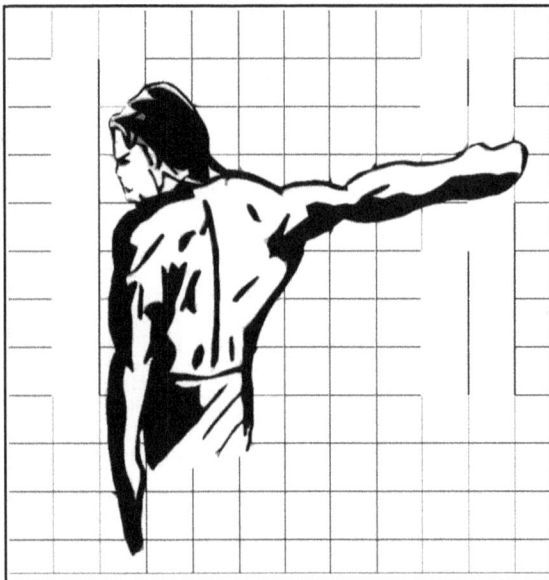

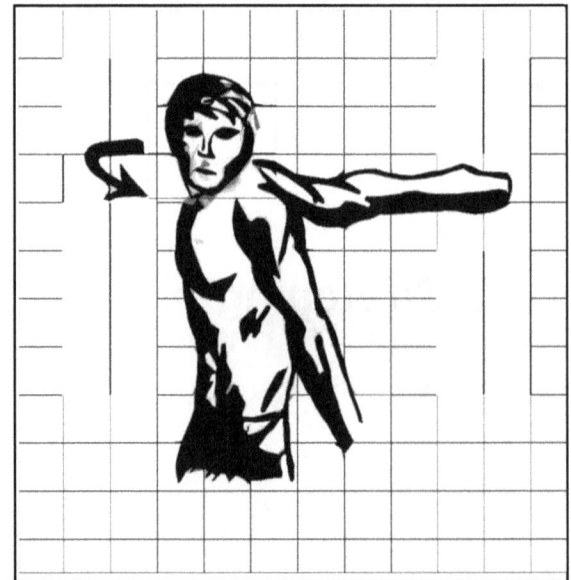

Lat stretch

In a standing position, face a wall and stretch your right arm across your chest, pointing toward the left corner of the ceiling. Hold for 15 to 30 seconds. Repeat procedure for left arm.

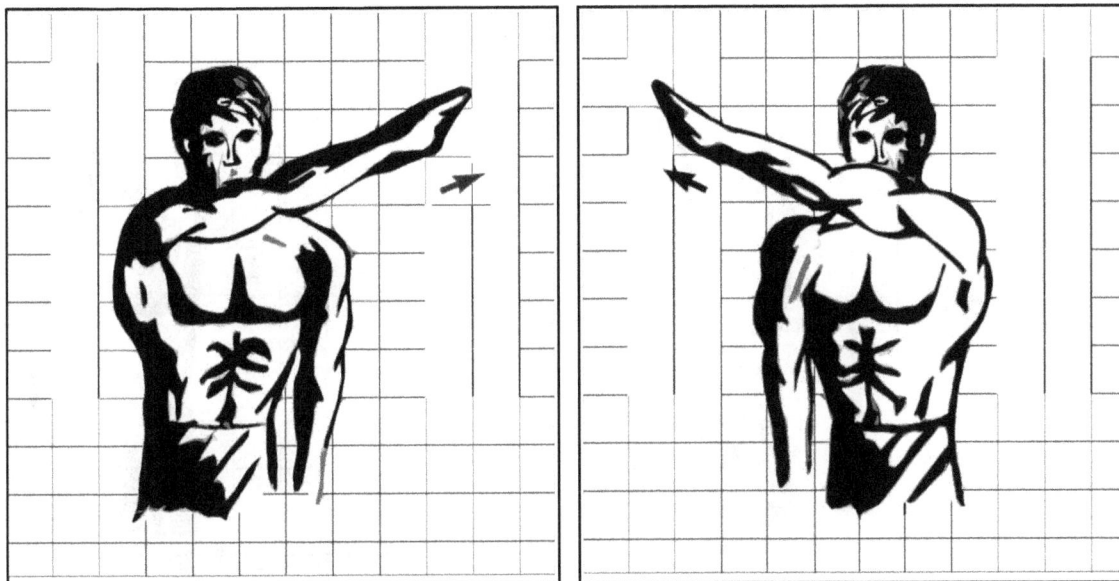

Side twists

Stand with your back towards a wall or fence at a distance of roughly 12 inches. Keeping your feet about shoulder width apart and your toes pointing straight, turn slowly to the right and touch the wall. Hold for 15 to 30 seconds. Repeat on left side.

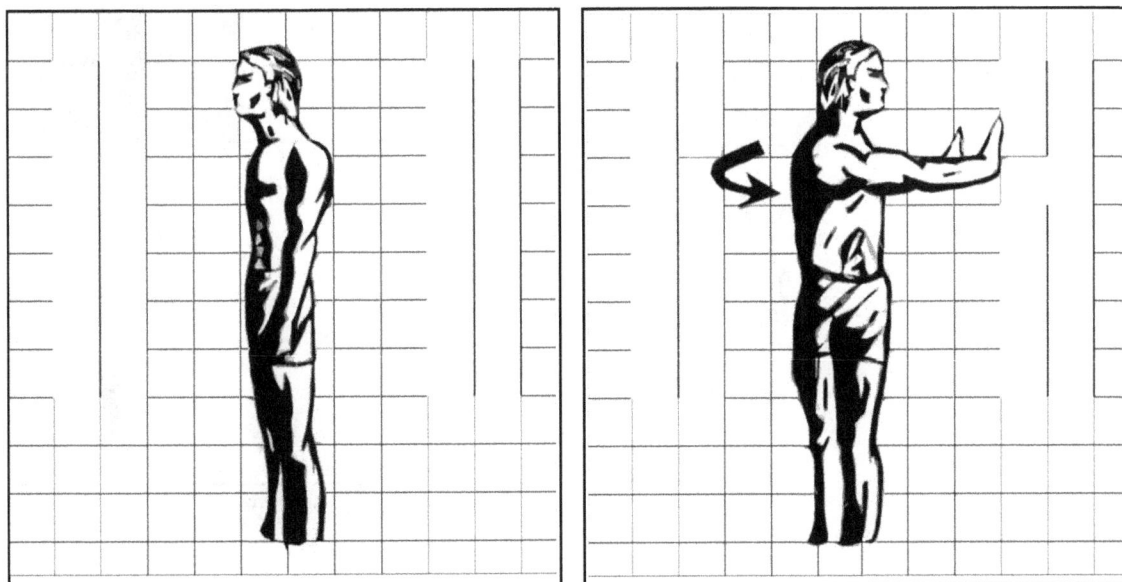

Hanging stretch

Hold on to a chin bar with both hands. Put your chin down and relax as you hang with your feet off the ground. Hold for 15 seconds. Gradually increase your time to 60 seconds.

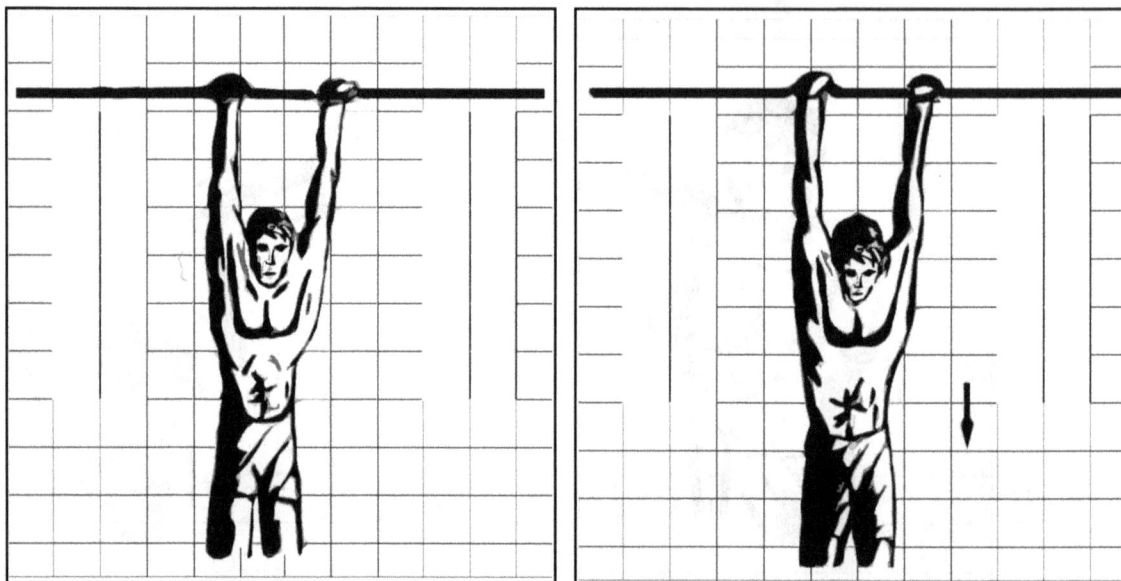

Quadriceps stretch

In a standing position, bend your right knee and grab your foot with your right hand. Try to touch your heal to your buttock. Hold for 15 to 30 seconds. Repeat for left leg.

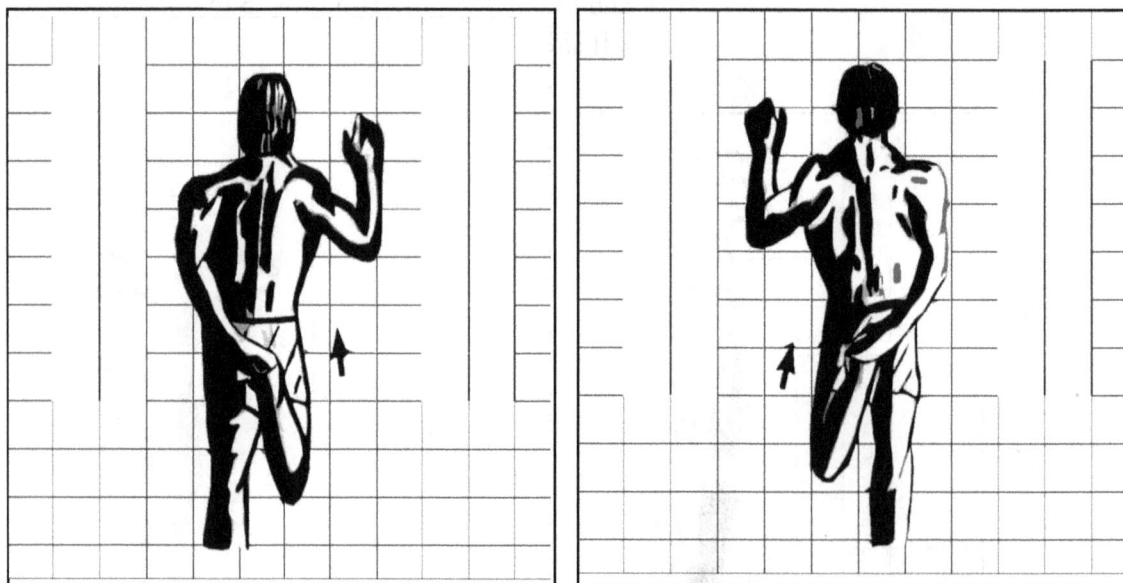

Hamstring stretch

While lying flat on your back, lift your right leg as high as possible without bending your knee. Grasp your leg with both hand and pull it back a bit further, enough so that you can feel tension but no any pain. Hold it there for 15 to 30 seconds. Repeat procedure for you left leg.

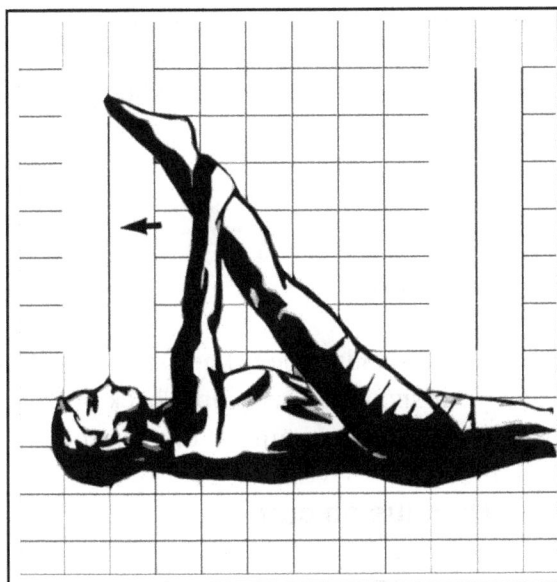

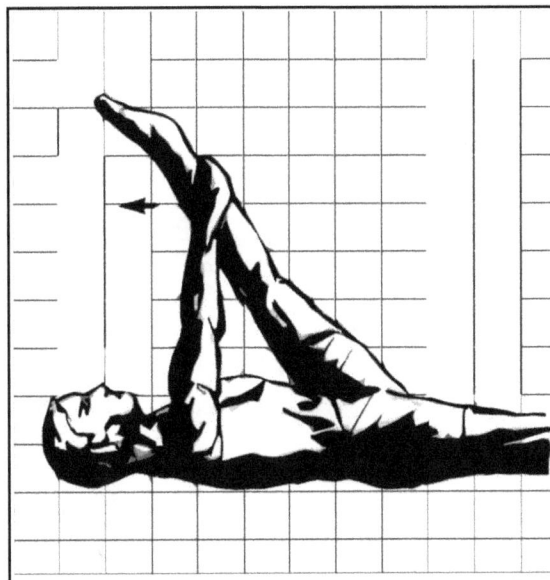

Groin stretch

While sitting on the floor with your feet a comfortable distance apart, lean forward from your hips. Do not lean forward from your head and shoulders. Keep your quadriceps relaxed and feet upright. Keep your hands out in front of you for balance and stability. Hold for 30 seconds.

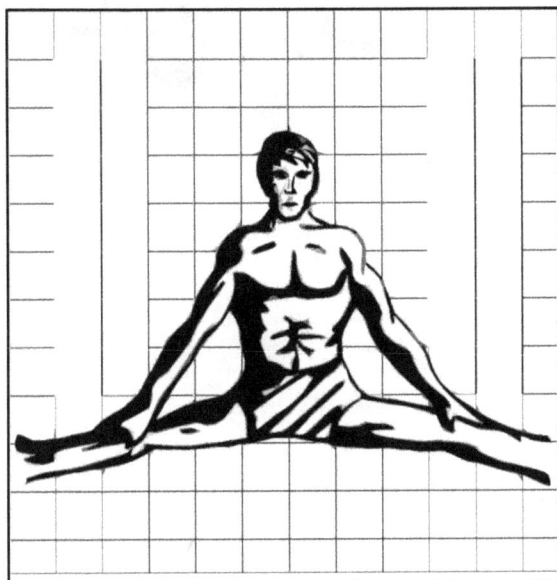

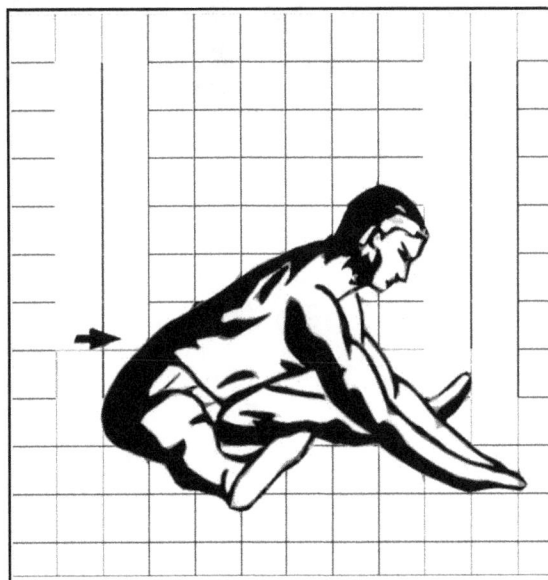

Resistance exercises

Examine the following exercises until you feel that you understand the basic movements. Although most of the illustrations are of movements performed with free weights, when ever possible, substitute the movement with it's Nautilus equivilent. If you choose to use free weights, make sure to train safe; For some exercises - like the bench press or behind neck press - it is essential that you have a training partner to remove the weight when you reach momentary muscular failure.

Abdominal crunch

While lying in the standard bent-knee sit-up position, very slowly raise your shoulders and upper back off the ground. Your lower back should remain flat on the ground. Lower yourself and repeat.
Alternate: Nautilus ab curl

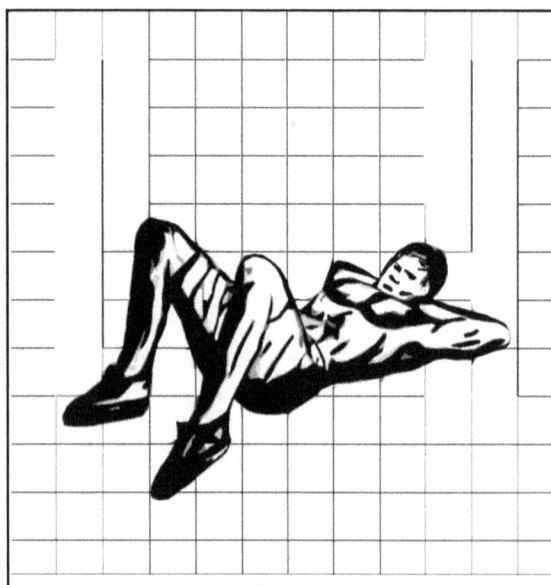

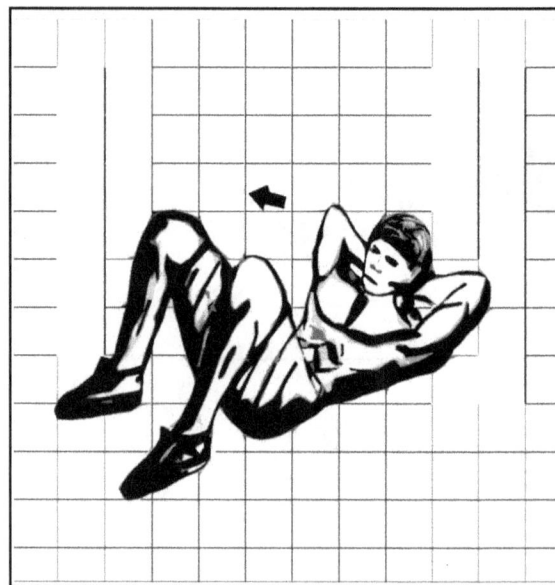

Barbell curl

In a standing position, hold the barbell with an underhand grip and curl it smoothly upward, keeping your back straight and your elbows at your sides. Lower the barbell and repeat.
Alternate: Nautilus bicep curl

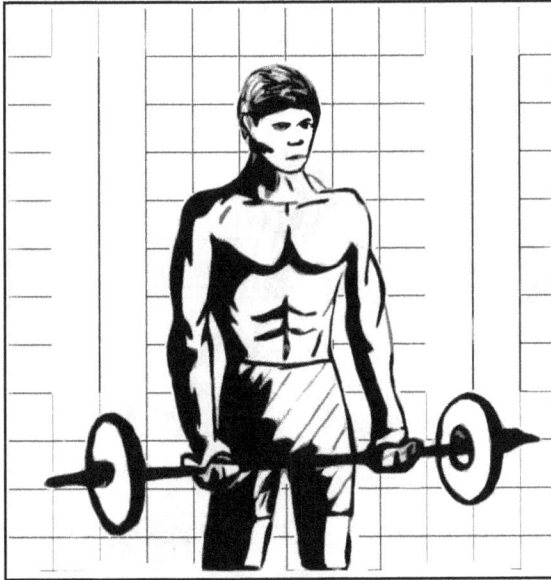

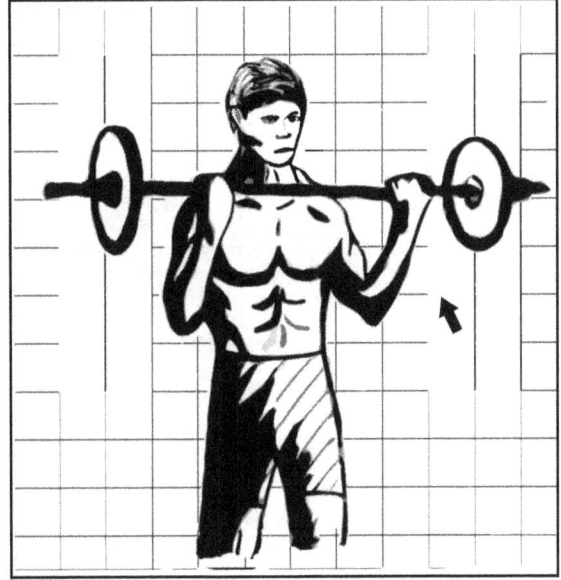

Barbell row

Place a barbell underneath a bench that is at least 20 inches high. Laying face down, grasp the barbell with an overhand grip and pull it up toward you until it hits the bottom of the bench. Lower and repeat.
Alternate: Nautilus row or low cable row

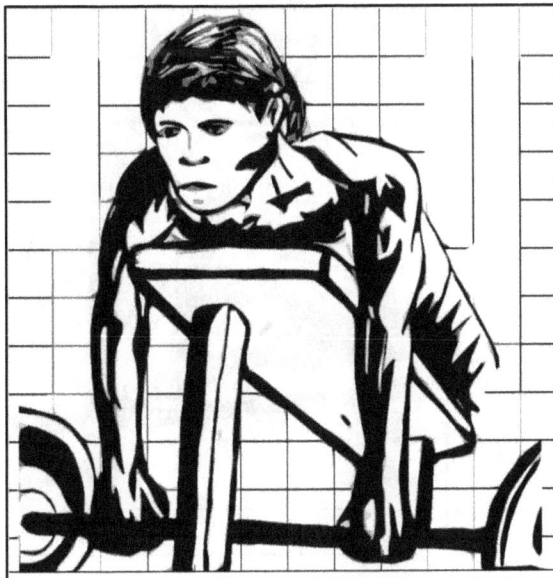

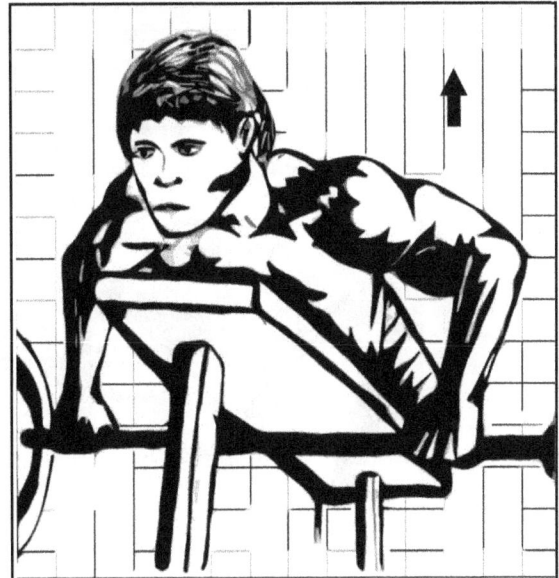

Behind- neck press

In a seated position, place the barbell behind your neck. Keeping your hand slightly wider than shoulder width, press the barbell smoothly overhead. Do not arch your back when performing this exercise.

Alternate: Nautilus shoulder press

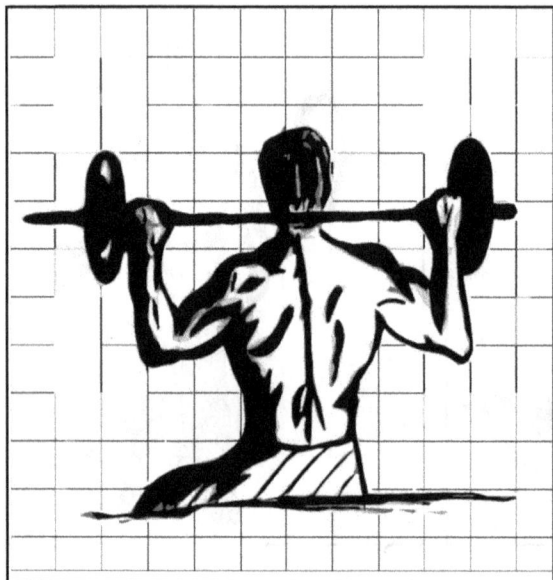

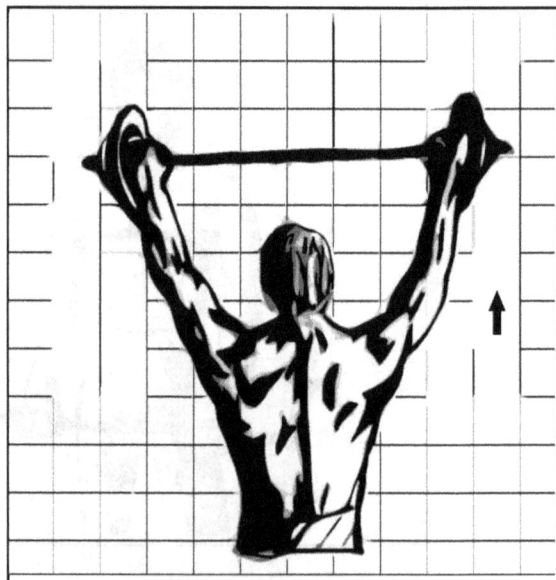

Bench press

Grasp the barbell at a wider than shoulder width and remove from the rack. Begin with the barbell touching your chest and press the barbell up until your elbows almost lock. Lower the barbell and repeat.

Alternate: Nautilus chest press

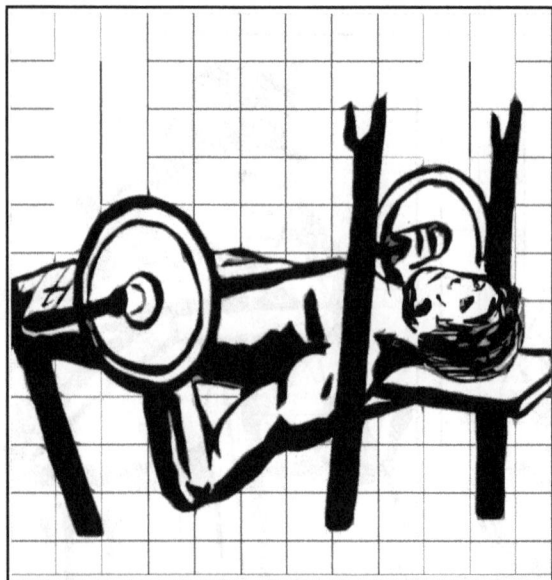

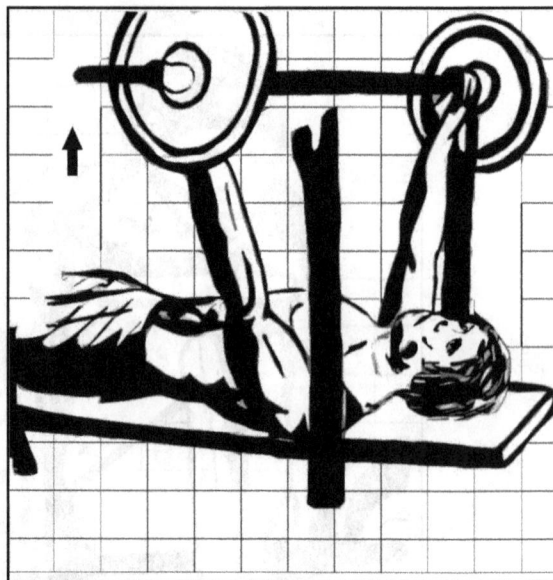

Bent-arm flyes

While lying on the bench, grasp two dumbbells and raise them slightly until they are at the same level as your chest. Bend your arms slightly and raise your arms above your chest, keeping arms bent.
Alternate: Nautilus pec deck

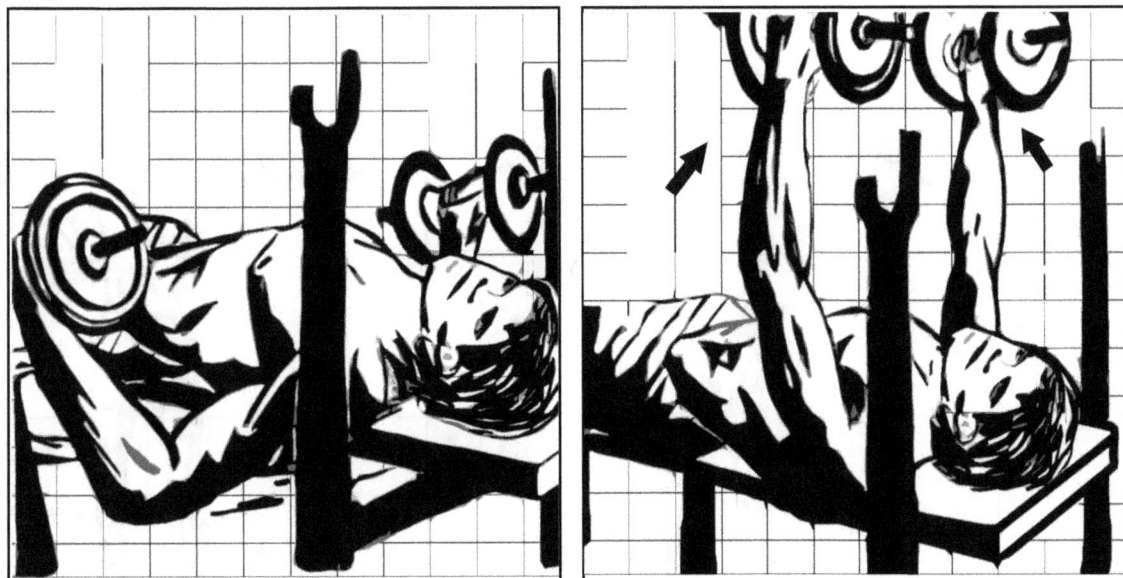

Bent-over raise

With knees slightly bent and a dumbbell in each hand, bend over at the waist, keeping your torso parallel to the floor. Raise each dumbbell until both arms parallel to the floor. Lower and repeat.

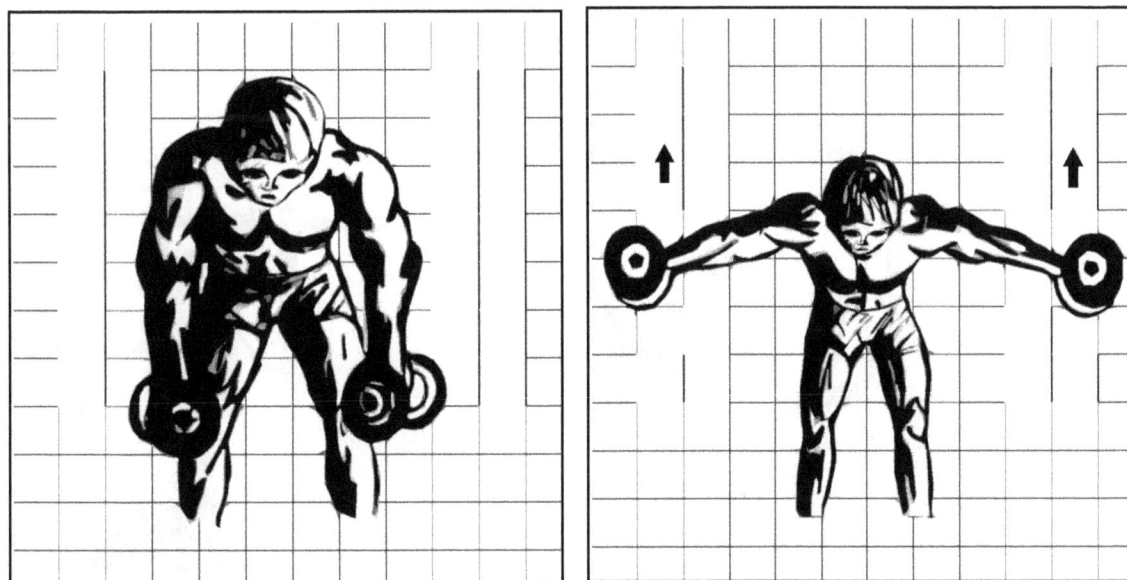

Calf Raise

Stand erect and place a barbell behind your neck and across your trapezius muscle. Keep your feet flat on the floor and shoulder width apart. Without bending your knees, try to stand up on your toes. Try to feel the muscle contract in your calves. Lower to the starting position and repeat.
Alternate: Calf machine

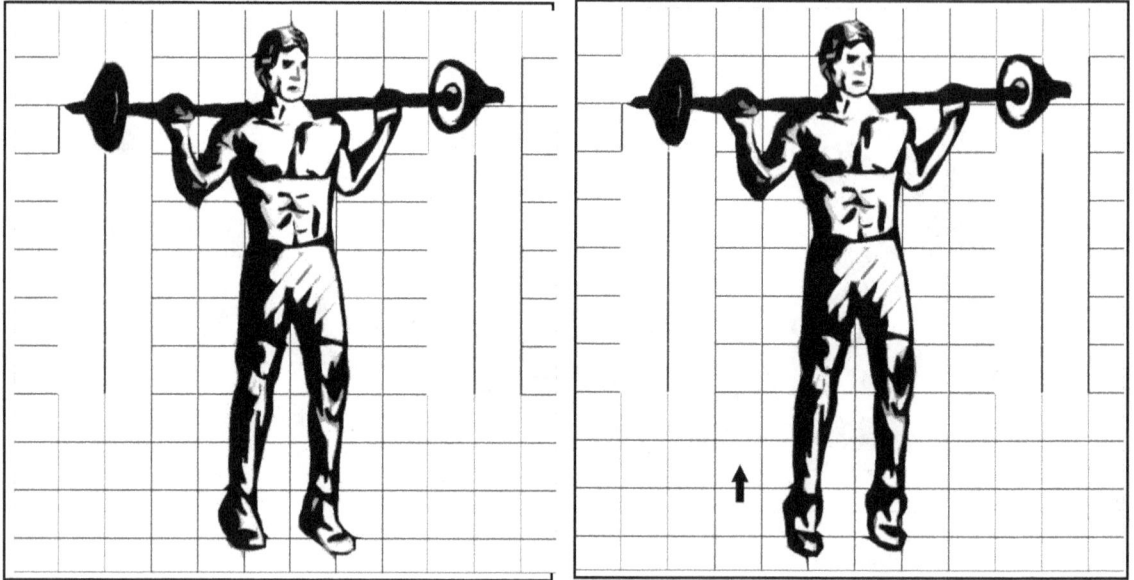

Chin-up

With an underhand grip, grasp a horizontal bar and hang. Your hands should be shoulder-width apart. Pull yourself up trying to touch the bar to your chest. Lower and repeat.

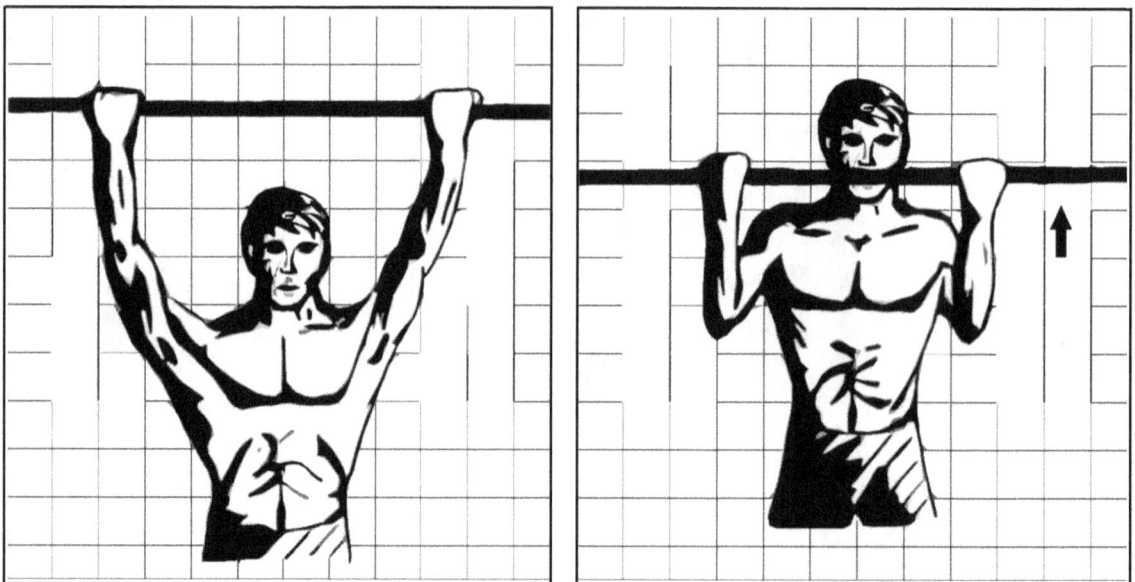

Hyper-extension

If possible, use a hyper-extension bench, otherwise, lay face down hanging over the end of a flat bench while someone holds your ankles. Lightly rest your hands behind your head and bend down at the waist. Slowly straighten your body up to starting position. Lower and repeat.

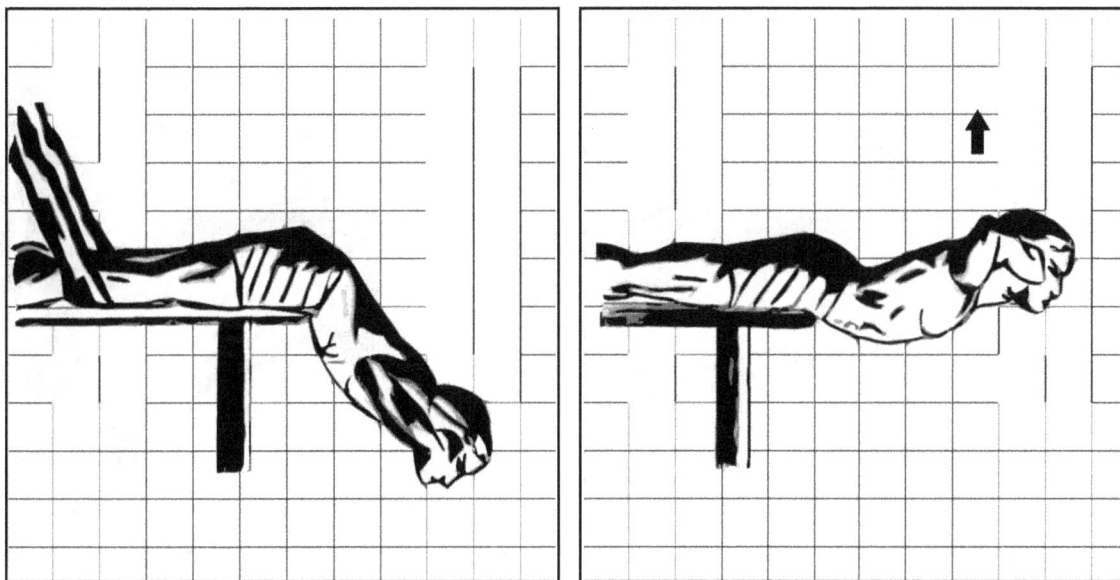

Lateral raise

With a dumbbell in each hand, stand straight with arms hanging at your sides. Raise your arms out straight from your   sides without bending your elbows until they are parallel with the floor. Lower slowly and repeat.

Alternate: Nautilus lateral raise

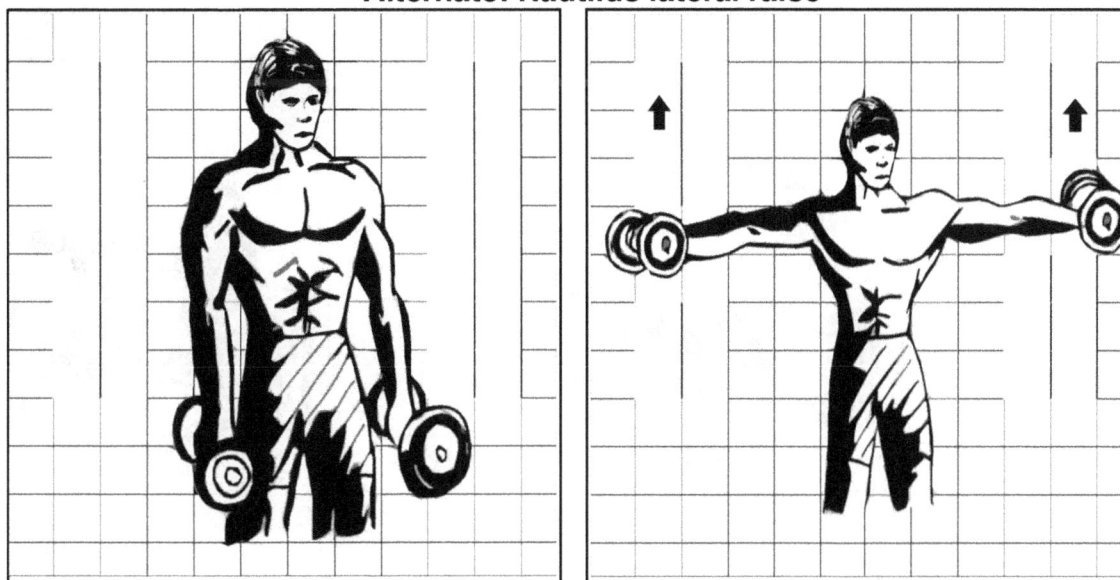

Leg Curl

Lay face down on the bench and place yor heels under the roller pads of the leg curl attachment. Bend your legs as far as possible. Pause in the top position. Lower and repeat.
Alternate: Nautilus leg curl

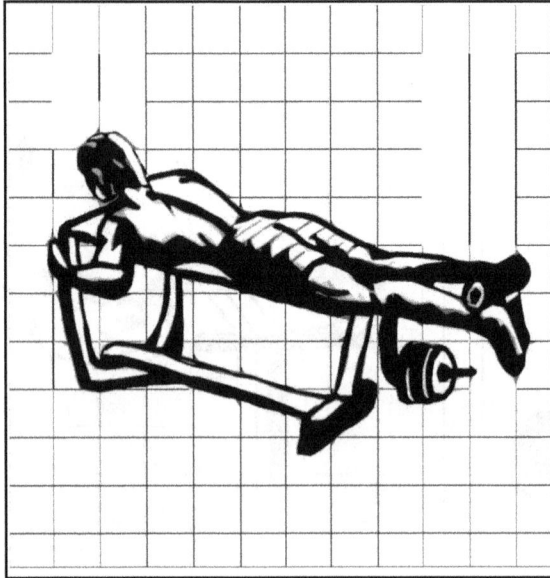

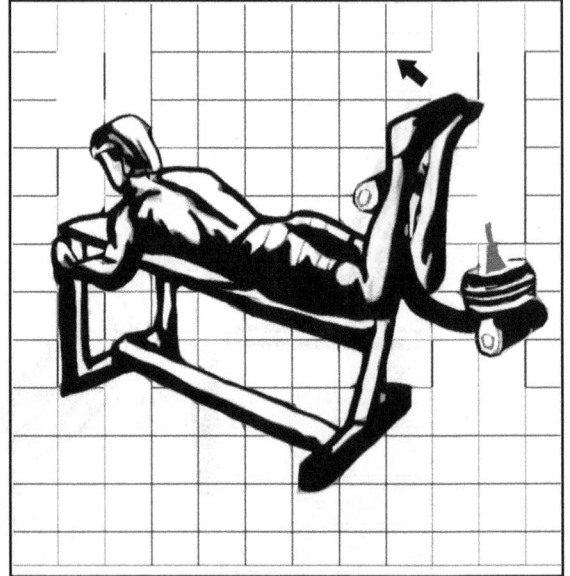

Leg extension

Sit on the end of the bench with your feet behind the roller pads of the leg extension attachment. Grasp the sides of the bench and smoothly straighten your legs. Pause in the top position. Lower and repeat.
Alternate: Nautilus leg extension

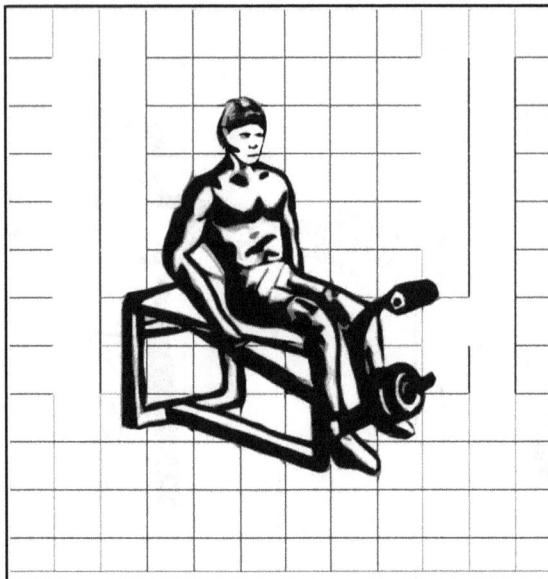

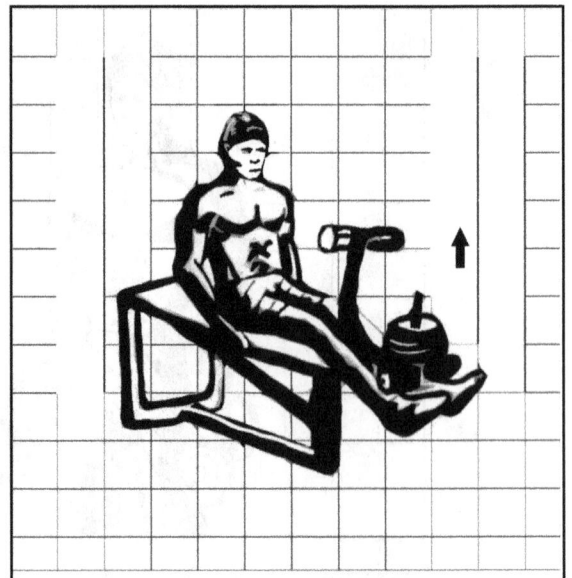

Overhead press

In a standing position, hold the barbell in front of your shoulders, palms facing outward, elbows bent. Keeping your hands shoulder-width apart, press the barbell overhead smoothly. Lower and barbell and repeat.
Alternate: Nautilus shoulder press

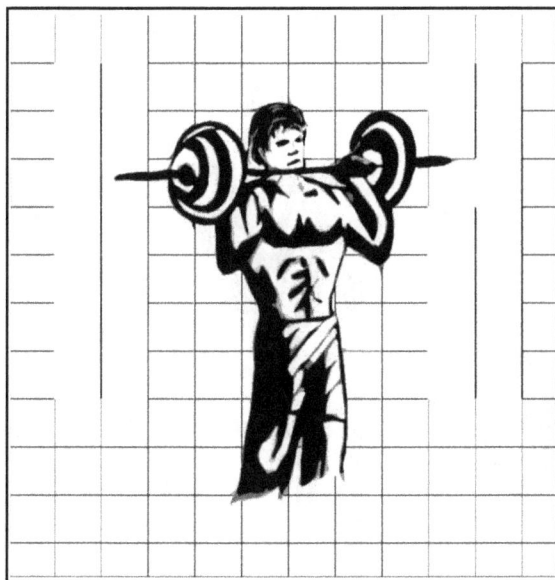

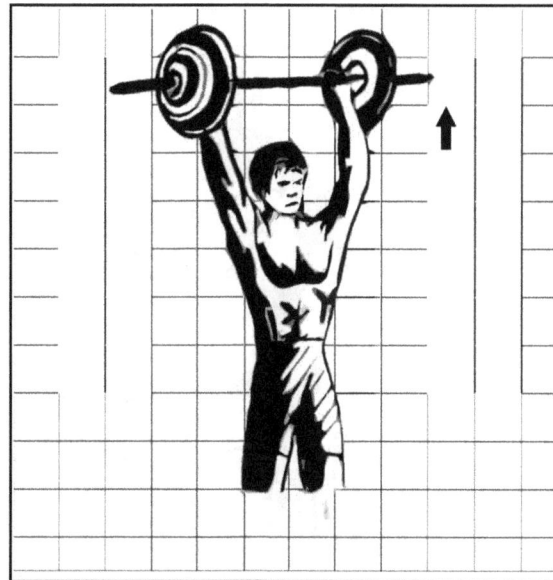

Parallel dip

Mount the parallel bars in the top position, keeping knees bent. Lower yourself, bending at the elbows. Raise yourself up to the top position and repeat.

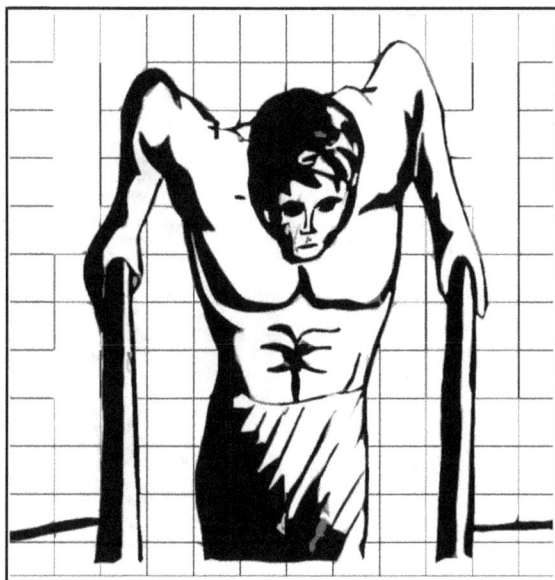

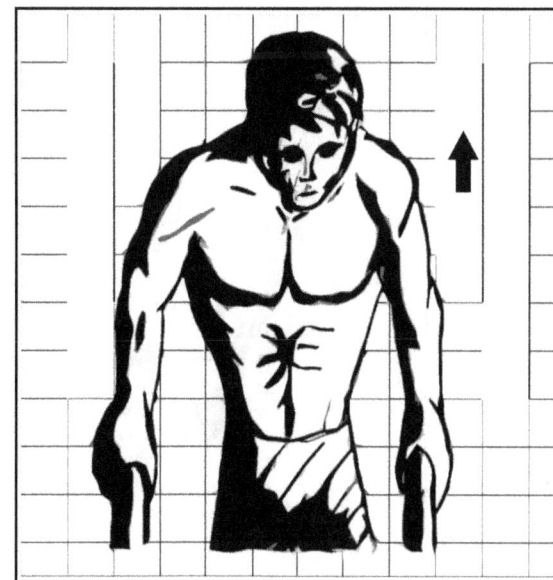

Preacher curl

While sitting in a preacher bench, grasp a barbell with an underhand grip and curl it towards you. Lower and repeat. Use about 25% less weight than you would normally use on the standing barbell curl.
Alternate: Nautilus bicep curl

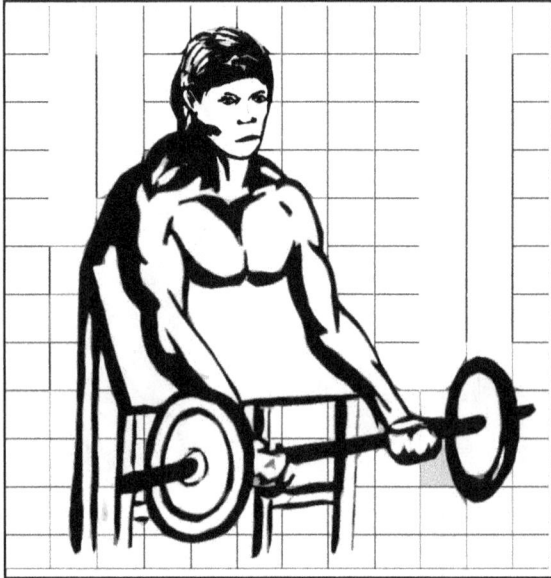

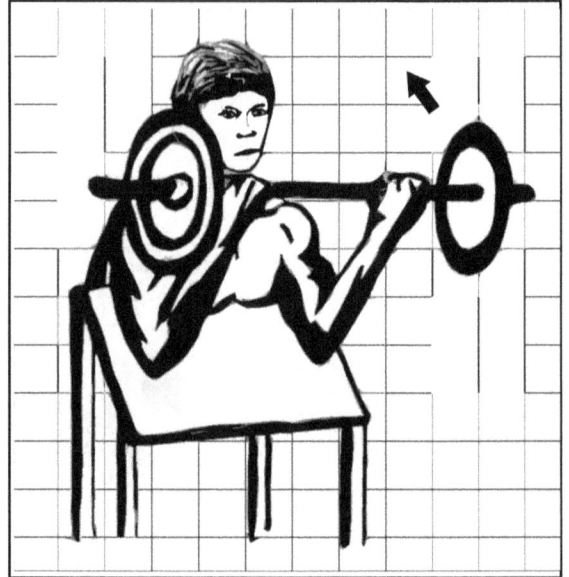

Pulldown behind neck

Grasp the pulldown bar with a grip that is slightly wider than shoulder-width. In a seated position, pull the bar smoothly behind your neck. Move back to the stretched position and repeat.

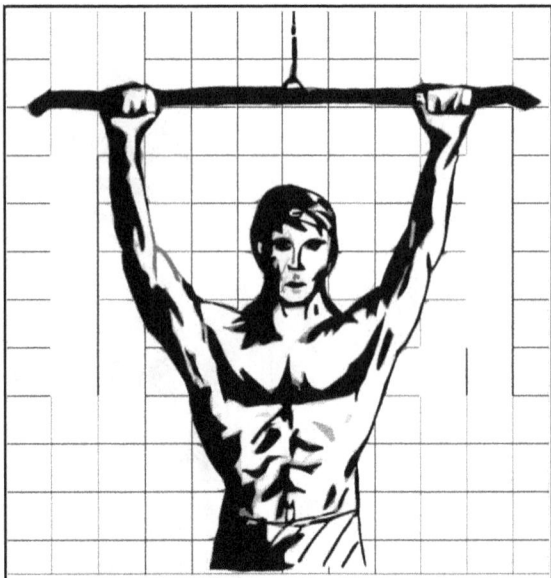

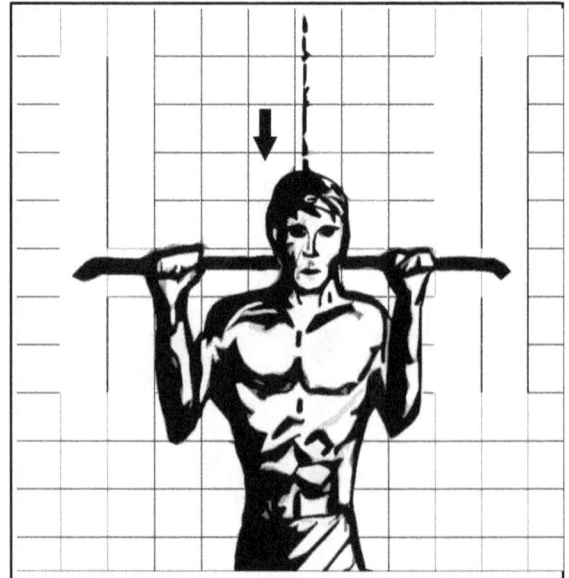

Pull-up

With an overhand grip, grasp a horizontal bar and hang.
Keep your hands slightly wider than shoulder width apart.
Pull yourself up and try to touch the bar to your chest.
Lower and repeat.

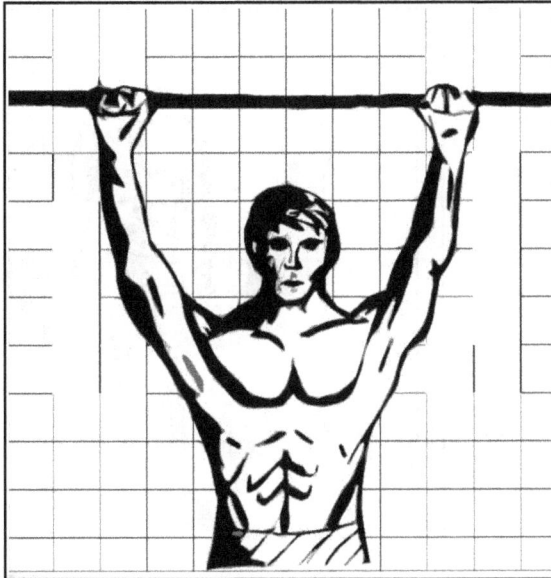

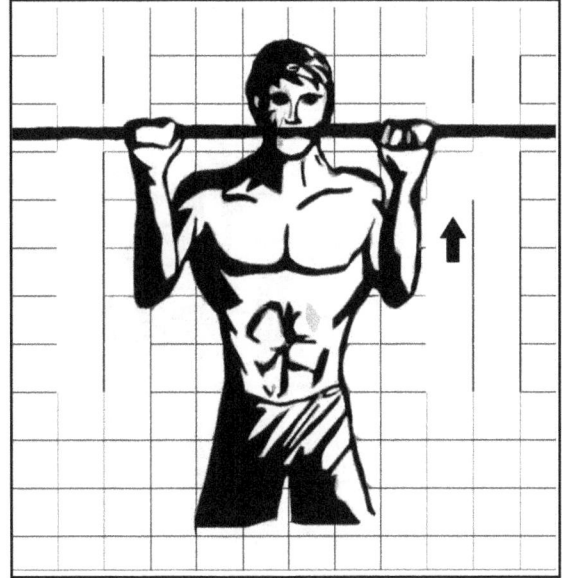

Push-up

Assume the classic push-up stance, keeping heand pointed
straight out, your body flat and parallel to the floor. Lower
yourself and repeat.

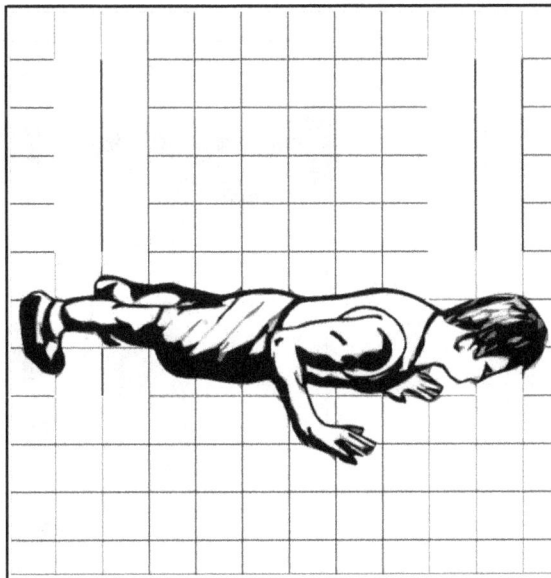

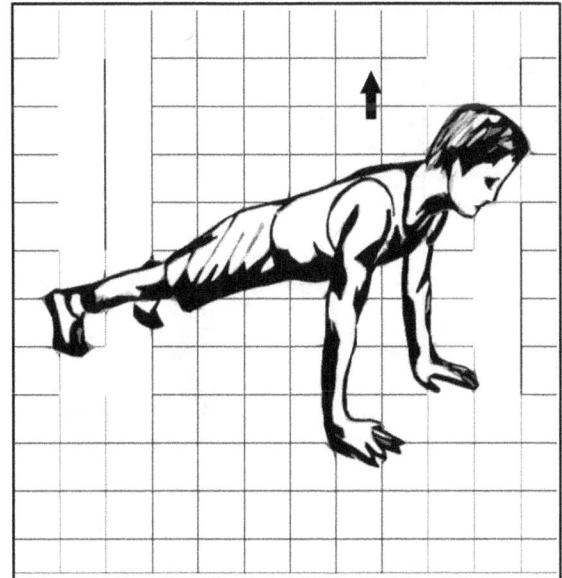

Reverse barbell shrug

In a standing position, place a barbell behind you and grasp it with an overhand grip. With arms straight, shrug your shoulders as high as possible. Lower and repeat.

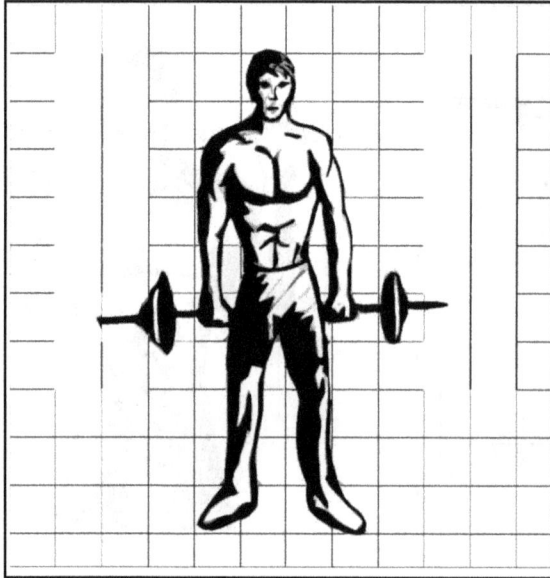

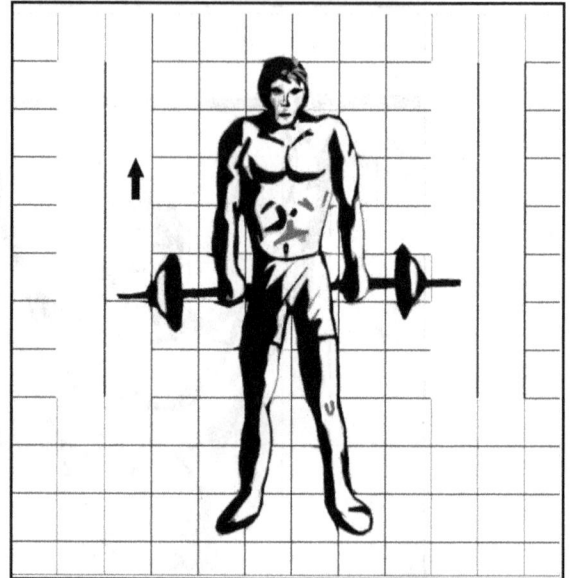

Squat

Stand erect and place a barbell behind your neck and across your trapezius muscle. Keep your feet shoulder width apart and head up at all times. Lower yourself, bending your knees and hips untill your thighs are parallel with the floor. Smoothly return to the standing position and repeat.
Alternate: Leg press

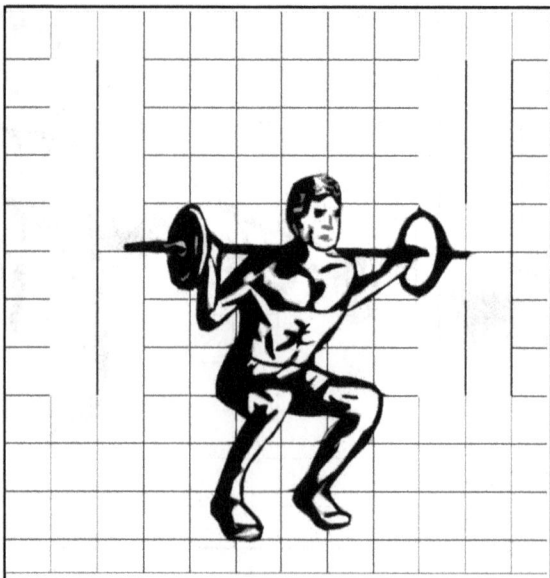

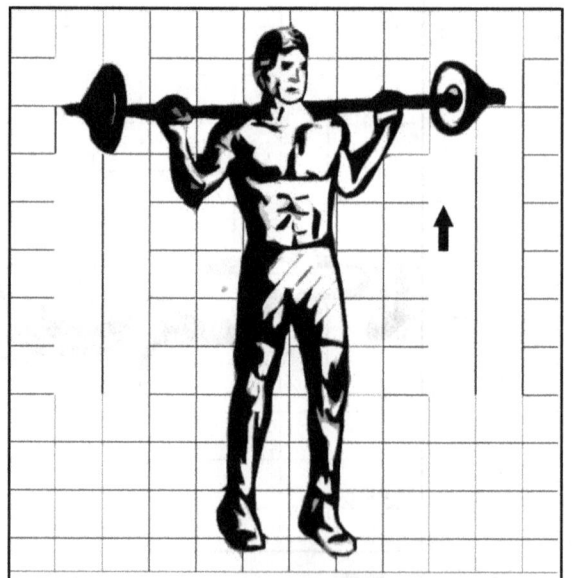

Stiff-legged deadlift

In a standing position, bend at the waist with knees locked and grasp the barbell. Lift to the top position. Lower and repeat.

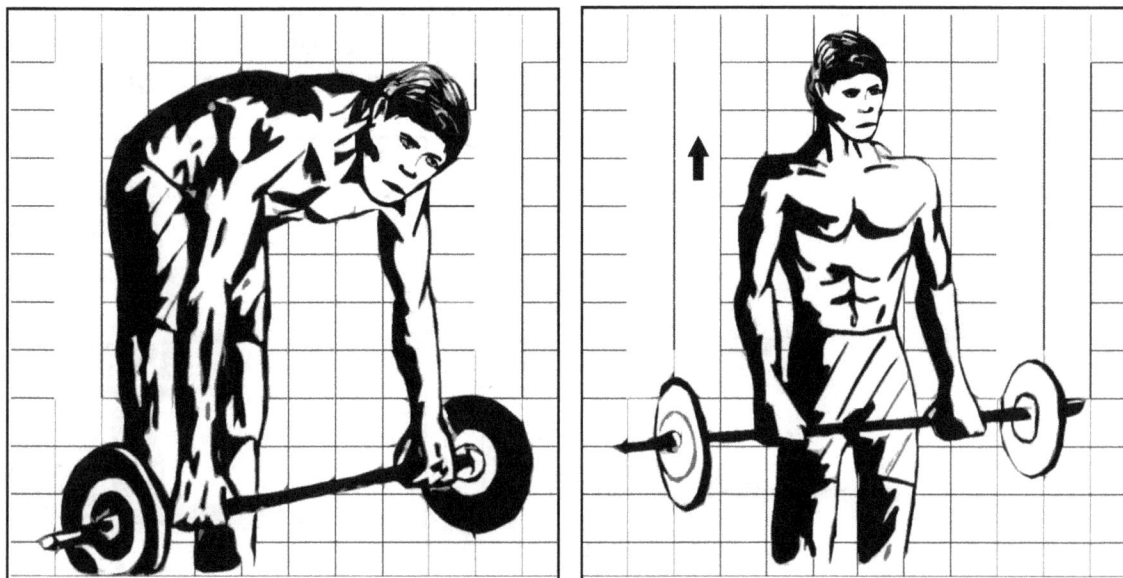

Straight arm pullover

Lay crossways to a flat bench with only shoulders and upper back touching while keeping your body straight. Grasp a light dumbbell on one end with both hands and hold it over your head with arms straight. Take a deep breath as you slowly lower the dumbbell behind your head, keeping your arms straight. Concentrate on the stretch at the bottom. Return to starting position and repeat.

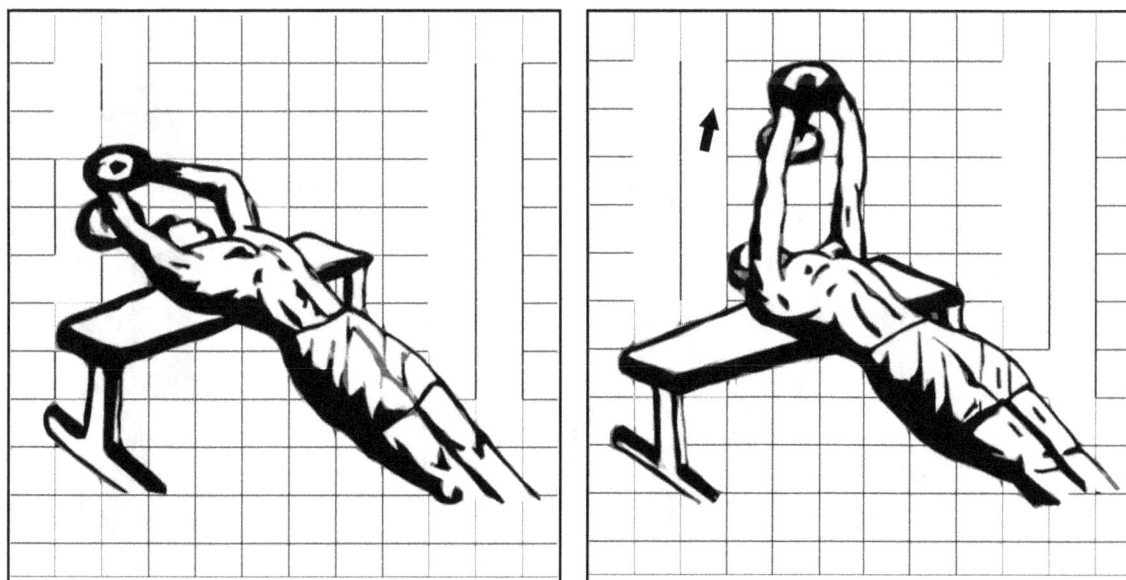

Tricep extension

While sitting on a bench, hold a dumbbell at one end with both hands behind your head. Press the dembbell overhead keeping your elbows close to your ears. Lower the dumbbell behind your head and repeat.
Alternate: Nautilus tricep extension

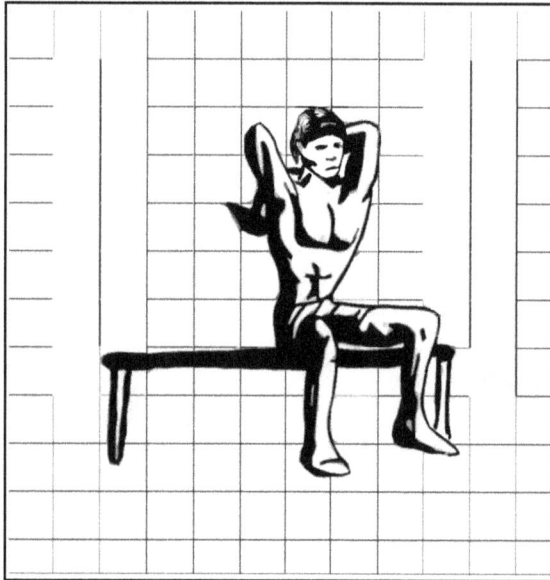

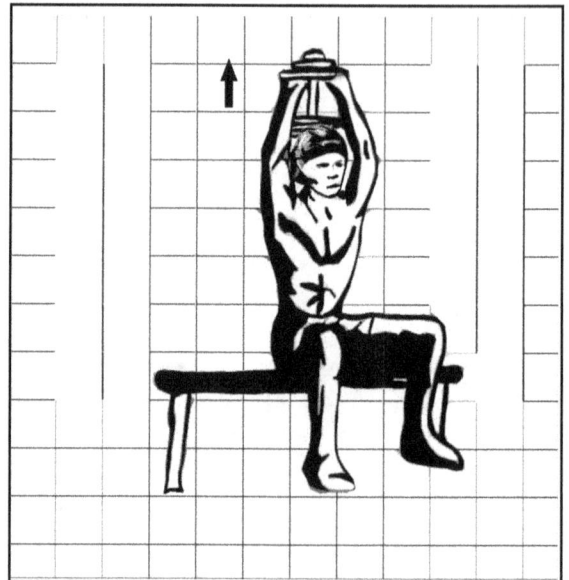

Upright row

In a standing position, grasp the barbell with an overhand grip, slightly wider than shoulder width. Pull the barbell up along your torso until it almost touches your neck. Pause, lower and repeat.

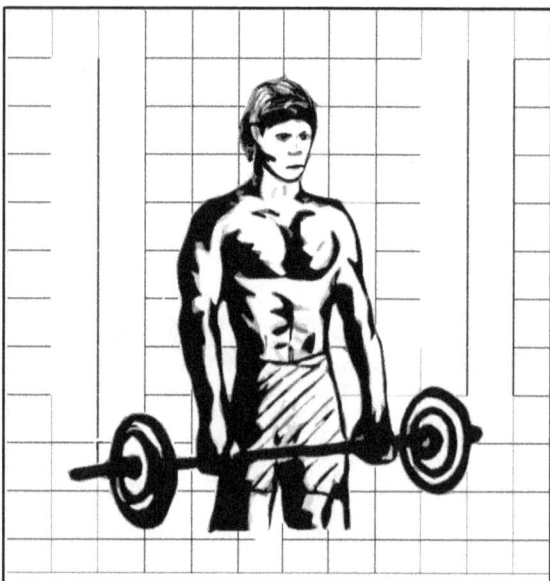

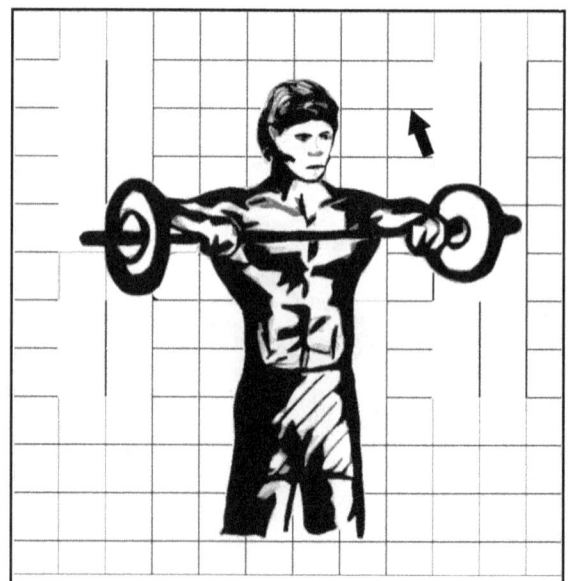

7 Putting It All Together

Frequency/length

When to work out

The fact that the body releases human growth hormone and other muscle repairing chemicals during sleep has led some to believe that working out later at night will achieve the best results. In theory, this makes sense, but for practical purposes, no particular time of day is *significantly* better than any other for working out, and the best time of day really all depends on your schedule. Some people prefer to workout after work, or even on their lunch break, while others like to get it over with in the morning. Wait an hour before or after meals, however, to prevent stomach upset. Also, avoid working out within 2 hours of bedtime, as it can interfere with sleep.

How often, how long

Allow at least 48 hours between workouts, and in some cases, up to 96 hours between an instense workout is necessary for muscles to completely recover. An ideal schedule for most would be; an intense weight training workout on Monday, an aerobic workout on Wednesday, and another intense weight training workout of Friday. Rest completely on the other days.
Your weight training workouts should not take more than 25-35 minutes to perform, while your Wednesday aerobic workout should be about 30 minutes. Try to leave no more than 1 minute of rest between sets during your weight training workouts.

Speed/cadence

Proper form

All exercises in this program, including stretches and those requiring repetitions, should be performed in a smooth, slow and controlled manner; As mentioned earlier, you should never jerk or toss a weight around. Sudden jerking or fast movements can lead to injury. During stretching movements, try to hold the stretched position for 5-10 seconds.

Repetitions

Except when utilizing certain specialized techniques, each repetition on every exercise should be performed in this manner: 2 to 3 seconds to lift the weight, pause 1 to 2 seconds in the contracted position, and lower the weight in 4 to 5 seconds.

Other considerations

Progression

As mentionied earlier, always remember to lift in a progressive manner; If your ideal repetition guideline were 8-12 repetitions, this means you choose a weight that allows you to perform only 8 repetions in good form. On your next workout, you must attempt to perform 9 or more repetitions with the same weight. When you can perform 12 repetitions with the same weight in good form, increase the weight by 5% and attempt 8 repetions with this new weight.

Focus

Focusing solely on the exercise at hand, and concentrating on each repetition is important for optimum results. By focusing on a muscles movement throughout the exercise, you can actually increase the intensity and therefore, your results.

Supplements

Of all the supplements mentioned in part one, a good, quality protein powder is the most important one recommended for this program. The other supplements can and do help, but a protein powder should be considered the cornerstone. This program will be effective without supplements, of course, but the addition of a good protein powder can make following a proper, balanced, effective diet much easier, and can improve your results tremendously. Just remember not to overdue it; never more than 20-30 grams of protein in one meal. If you are interested in trying some of the other supplements mentioned in this book, they should be taken in the following doses:

Creatine monohydrate

Loading Phase(first 5-7 days):
Creatine should be mixed with a high GI beverage such as gatorade, fruit juice or even sugar water.

189 pounds or under: 20 grams per day
190 pounds to 220:   25 grams per day
221 pounds and above: 30 grams per day

Maintenance Phase(after 5-7 days of loading):

All weights: 5 grams per day

Always remember to drink plenty of water while supplementing with creatine; 1/2 to 1 gallon per day.

L-arginine

1,000 mg - 2,000 mg   3x per day with meals

L-theanine

100 mg - 200 mg   30 minutes before and after workout

L-tyrosine

1,500 mg - 3,000 mg 30 minutes before workout

Methoxyisoflavone

200 mg - 400 mg 2x per day

Myostatin blockers

Myostatin blockers containing Cystoseira canariensis extract:

500 mg 2x per day

Phosphatidylserine

400 - 1,200 mg 30 minutes before workout

ZMA

For men;
30 mg zinc/450 mg magnesium/10.5 mg B6 at bedtime

For women
20 mg zinc/300 mg magnesium/7 mg B6 at bedtime

Building a routine

Some people find that when a lot of information is presented to them all at once, they hardly know where to start, and it is all too easy to forget important points along the way. If you find yourself experiencing this same problem, one of the best remedies is to establish a routine that incorporates all the major points, so that it eventually becomes habit. Experts say that it takes three weeks for a routine to become habit. Once that habit is established, very little conscious effort or memory recall is necessary. It becomes second nature - just a normal part of your daily routine.

Points to remember

There are several major points that must be remembered in order for your training to be effective. Write each of these down by hand in a list, or make a copy of the following pages, and try to incorporate them into your daily routine. At first, you may need to take this list with you, but in a few weeks you will have established these points as habit;

Before working out:

√ Take phosphatidylserine, 400 mg - 1,200 mg

√ Take L-tyrosine, 1,500 - 3,000 mg

√ Take L-theanine, 100-200 mg

√ Stretch

√ Warm up with 15-20 minutes of aerobic activity

√ Visualize

√ Evaluate yourself

When working out:

√ Lift weight in 2 seconds, hold for 2, lower in 4 seconds

√ Sip a high GI beverage, such as Gatorade, *during* your workout.

√ Take every set to momentary muscular failure.

√ Use a training partner or "spotter" if possible

√ Use proper form - perform repetitions smoothly

√ Try to avoid "locking out" in the extended position of a repetition

When working out(continued):

√ Follow your ideal repetions guideline(see chapter 8)

√ In most cases, perform only 1 set of each exercise

√ Be progressive; always attempt either more weight or more repetitions

√ Keep rest between sets to a maximum of 1 minute

√ Except during specialized routines, exercise largest muslces first

√ For safety and variety, substitute Nautilus machines for free weights whenever possible

√ Keep accurate records to measure your progress

√ Focus

√ During aerobic work, watch your heart rate

After working out:

√ Drink high GI drink with 15-30 grams of protein within 30 minutes after workout

√ Stretch

√ Try electro-muscle stimulation

√ Rest

√ Take 100 mg - 200 mg L-theanine

Throughout your day:

√ Choose foods with a low GI value

√ Eat a variety of fruits, vegetables , whole grains and lean protein.

Throughout your day(continued):

√ Remember that a serving size is about as big as a deck of cards

√ Eat 5-6 small meals, instead of 3 big ones - eat every 2-3 hours to keep blood sugar stable

√ Drink plenty of water - 6-8 ounces every 2 hours

√ Take a multi-vitamin with no more than 100% RDA

√ Visualize your fitness goals

√ When cravings come, remember your cheat day

√ Learn lucid dreaming; test your state

√ Try self-hypnosis, meditation and other mind/body techniques

√ Keep your meals balanced

√ Take Methoxyisoflavone, Myostatin blocker, L-arginine Creatine monohydrate supplements

√ Take a nap, if possible

At bedtime:

√ Take ZMA supplement

√ Get plenty of sleep. 7-10 hours, if possible.

√ Pray

√ Visualize

√ Rest and relax

8 Preliminaries

Before beginning this exercise program, there are several things that should be done first:

Consult your Doctor

Exercise, especially high-intensity weight training, can be dangerouse for some people. Existing conditions, such as asthma, high blood pressure, diabetes, etc. can be aggravated by exercise of any kind. For people with these or other pre-existing conditions, it is essential to consult with a doctor before beginning this or any other exercise program. Regardless of your condition, it is always a good idea to have a physical before embarking on a new exercise program, particularly if you are over the age of 35 and have risk factors such as; a family history of heart disease, you are a smoker, or lead a mostly sedentary lifestyle.

Evaluate your body

A thorough evaluation of the existing condition of your body can help you determine your progress throughout the program, and make necessary adjustments along the way to meet your goals. It is easy sometimes to forget the condition you were in when you started, and to ignore small, gradual improvements along the way. Keeping accurate records of the changes in your body can remind and encourage you, and is essential for continued motivation and ultimate success. Consider the following when determining your current condition, and deciding on your fitness goals;

Bodyweight

Don't get too hung up on your weight, as it is not always the best way to evaluate your physique; a number of factors can determine bodyweight; fat to muscle ratio, bone density, water retention. Use it as a *very general* guide to where you are physically, and where you want to be. Record your weight in the chart provided at the end of this chapter(Figure A).

Body measurements

An excellent way to chart your bodysculpting progress is with careful circumference measurements of your body using a tape measure. Some measurements will be difficult and possibly inaccurate if taken by yourself, so consider having a friend or training partner assist you. All measurements should be taken "cold", that is, before working out, without a muscle "pump". The tape should be pulled tight *against* the skin, but not so tight that it presses *into* the skin. Measure the following areas in the manner described, and record them in the chart provided at the end of this chapter (Figure B):

Calves

Stand up straight with your feet flat on the floor. Do not tighten or flex your calves. Measure each calf at the largest point.

Thighs

Again, stand up straight with your feet flat on the floor. Try to relax your thighs as much as possible. Measure each thigh just below the buttock.

Hips

Stand up straight, both feet flat, as before. Try to distribute your weight equally on both legs. Stretch the tape around the hips at the largest point of the buttocks.

Waist

While standing up straight, try to keep your abdomen in it's normal state; that is, do not suck it in, or relax it excessively. Take the measurement at the level of the belly button.

Chest

Stand up straight and relax. Do not spread your lats or inflate your lungs. Breathe in and exhale halfway. Take measurements at the level of your nipples. Make sure the tape is straight across your back and at the same level as the front.

Forearms

Keeping your arm straight, make a fist and flex your forearm muscle. Do not bend the elbow or the wrist. Measure at the largest point below the elbow.

Upper arms

Raise your arm up to shoulder height and bend at the elbow, flexing your biceps in the classic body builder pose. Measure your arm at the largest point. The tape measure should be at a right angle to the arm bone.

Neck

Keep your chin up and your eyes looking forward. Relax your neck. Take the measurement an inch or so below the chin.

Bodyfat

The best way to measure body fat is with a pair a skinfold calipers; a pair of specially designed calipers are used to measure folds of skin and underlying fat at various points on the body. These can be tricky to use, however, and sometimes difficult to find. If you can find one, or can have a qualified professional perform the test for you, it is probably the most accurate way to obtain a bodyfat percentage reading - outside of expensive body density tests performed in water tanks. There are a couple of other easier, but less accurate methods for measuring bodyfat; while these methods may not be as accurate, they are still useful for monitoring your progress; Try one or both of these techniques and record your results in the chart provided(Figure C).

Skinfold pinch

1. With the help of a friend, find the area midway between your rear shoulder and your elbow on the back of your arm. At this point, have your friend pinch a double layer of skin and underlying adipose(fat) tissue between his thumb and forefinger. Be sure not to pinch any

muscle tissue, only fat and skin. Try to pull the skin and fat away from the muscle. A quick, temporary flexing of the triceps muscle, if necessary, can help in the process of seperating muscle from skin and fat.

2. Using a ruler, measure the thickness of skin and fat(in millimeters). Try not to press the ruler against the skin when taking this measurement.

3. Wait 2 seconds and take the measurement again.

4. Add the two measurements together and then determine the average.

When finished, refer to the chart below to determine your bodyfat percentage, and record your results in the chart provided at the end of the chapter(Figure C).

Bodyfat percentage

Triceps Skin Pinch (mm)	% Bodyfat(men)	% Bodyfat(women)
6	5-9	8-13
13	9-13	13-18
19	13-18	18-23
25	18-22	23-28
38	22-27	28-33

Biceps measurment

Another method for keeping track of changes in body fat is to simply measure the difference between your relaxed bicep and flexed bicep; The greater the difference in circumference, the greater the fat loss. While this method won't give you a bodyfat percentage rate, it will help you to track changes in bodyfat quickly and easily:

1. Let your arm hang relaxed at your side. Wrap a tape

measure around your arm at the largest point. Record the measurement on the chart provided.

2.   Raise your arm up to shoulder height and bend at the elbow, flexing your bicep. Make sure to take your measurement at the same point as the relaxed measurement. Write down the results.

3.   Record the difference between the relaxed and flexed bicep in the chart.

Before and after photos

Have you ever had the experience of seeing a friend or relative for the first time in a year or two, and being amazed at how much they had changed? Chances are, those that have seen your friend on a day to day basis, and perhaps your friend himself, didn't notice any significant changes at all. The fact is, small, gradual changes are rarely noticed, and it is easy to forget what we looked like just a short time ago - whether it be a few years, a few months or a few weeks. That's why taking photographs before starting any body sculpting program can be one of the best methods for measuring progress and producing motivation; At the end of eight weeks, you might not think you have made much progress, but a simple comparison of before and after photo graphs can reveal the truth of the matter, and motivate you to continue in your exercise and bodysculpting pursuits. We have all seen the dramatic before and after pictures from those physique transformation contests. Sometimes the changes seen are truly incredible. Let's start recording *your* incredible transformation right now:

1.   Start by finding an uncluttered, neutral colored background. Hang a white sheet behind you, if necessary.

2.   Dress in shorts or a bathing suit, revealing as much of your body as possible(while still remaining tasteful!)

3.   Make sure the lighting is correct; bright, natural light focused directly on you is best. Avoid heavy shadows, or overly dark areas.

4.   Try to take at least six photos: front relaxed, back relaxed, right side relaxed, left side relaxed, and a couple fully flexed poses of your choice, such as; double biceps

flex(the classic "muscle man" pose), ab flex pose or the "lat" spread. Be creative. Any poses that show the major muscle groups are good choices.

5. Paste the before photos in the spaces provided in chapter 15(Evaluation) of this book.

Strength/ neurological efficiency

As mentioned earlier, neurological efficiency is a person's ability to recruit muscle fibers; the more efficient a person's neuro-muscular system, the more muscle fibers he can recruit at one time. Testing your neurological efficiency can help determine the ideal repetition scheme for your body- one that will stimulate growth most effectively based on your own neuromuscular system.

To determine your neurological efficiency and the ideal number of repetitions for your training use the following procedure:

For upper body:

1. Start by warming up with the biceps curl; choose a weight that will allow you to perform 10-15 repetitions in very strict form. Stop short of momentary muscular failure.

2. Rest 3-5 minutes.

3. On the biceps curl, choose a weight that will only allow

    you to perform 1 repetition in good form. This is inherently dangerous - so be careful to avoid jerking or "throwing" the weight around. Perform the repetition with strict, controlled movement, and stop immediately if you experience any pain.

4. Rest 2 minutes.

5. Take 80% of your one repetion maximum weight, and perform as many repetions as possible in good form.

When you can no longer perform a strict repetition, stop.

6. Refer to the repetition chart provided to find out your ideal number of repetitions.

    Use the same number of repetitions discovered for biceps curl for all other single-joint, "isolation" exercises for the upper body, such as; triceps extension, shoulder raises, reverse barbell shrug, etc. For upper body exercises involving multiple joints, such as; bench press, overhead press, or pulldown behind neck, add 2 repetions to the low and high ends of this number. Record your results in the repetition guide(figure D).

For lower body:

1. Start by warming up on the leg extension; choose a weight that will allow you to perform 10-15 repetitions in very strict form. Stop short of momentary muscular failure.

2. Rest 3-5 minutes.

3. On the leg extension, choose a weight that will only allow you to perform 1 repetition in good form. This is inherently dangerous - so be careful to avoid jerking or "throwing" the weight around. Perform the repetition with strict, controlled movement, and stop immediately if you experience any pain.

4. Rest 2 minutes.

5. Take 80% of your one repetion maximum weight, and perform as many repetions as possible in good form. When you can no longer perform a strict repetition, stop.

6, Refer to the repetition chart provided to find out your ideal number of repetitions.

Use the same number of repetitions discovered for leg extensions for all other single-joint, "isolation" exercises for the lower body, such as; leg curl and calf raise. For lower body exercises involving multiple joints, such as; squats and deadlifts, add 2 repetions on the low and high ends to this number. Record your results in the repetition guide provided(figure D).

Bodyweight (figure A)

Date	Weight in pounds

Body measurements (figure B)

Circumference (in inches)

Right Calve	
Left Calve	
Right Thigh	
Left Thigh	
Hips	
Waist	
Chest	
Right Forearm	
Left Forearm	
Right Upper Arm	
Left Upper Arm	
Neck	

Bodyfat measurement (Figure C)

Triceps skinfold (mm)	Bodyfat %

Relaxed bicep (mm)	Flexed bicep (mm)	Difference

Strength test sheet

Biceps curl	Leg extension

Weight (1 repetition max.)

Weight (80% of 1 repetition max.)

# of repetitions with 80% of 1 rep. max

Ideal repetitions chart

Number of repetitions(w/80%max)	Ideal repetition range
1	1-2
2	1-3
3	2-4
4	3-5
5	4-6
6	5-7
7	6-8
8	7-9
9	8-10
10	8-12
11	9-13
12	10-14
13	11-15
14	12-16
15	13-17
16	14-18
17	14-20
18	15-21
19	16-22
20	17-23
21	18-24

Ideal repetitions guide (figure D)

Upper body (single joint)   **Upper body (single joint)**

Lower body (multiple joint)   **Lower body (multiple joint)**

Part Three

The 8-Week Total Body Makeover

9 Laying the foundation: Weeks 1-3

Pouring the the concrete

Most architects would agree that the first step to building any great structure is building a good, solid foundation. Before building anything else, they must pour the concrete and set the foundation. Similarly, in order to gain muscular size in the most efficient manner, you must first concentrate on building strength in a few basic exercises - nothing fancy until a foudation of muscle mass has been attained.

Almost all great bodybuilders - from Steve Reeves to Arnold Shwartzenegger - started out with the basics, and you should too. Concentration on a few basic multiple joint movements now will result in awesome gains in overall size and strength and prepare you for more advanced techniques later on down the road.

The first two exercises for this routine have been arranged to stimulate growth hormone release and rib cage expansion; You will be performing two sets of the squat and the straight arm pullover. The first set should consist of 15 to 20 repetitions of "breathing" squats, immediately followed by 15 to 20 repetitions of straight-arm pullovers. As mentioned earlier, "Breathing" squats consist of perfoming 10 repetions in the normal manner,and beginning with the eleventh repetition, taking 2 or 3 deep breaths between repetitions.

Start out by choosing a weight that will allow you to perform 15 repetitions. When you can perform 20 or more repetitions with the same weight, increase the weight by 5%. The straight-arm pullover should be performed in the same manner. Do not allow more than 10 seconds between the two exercises, and do not apply any special techniques, such as progressive negative tension, forced reps, etc. On the second set, both exercises should be perfomed in the regular manner, using your individual repetitions guideline for lower and upper body. Also, remember to watch your diet; keep track of what you are putting into your body - it will be easier to remember and adjust if you write it down. Try to follow the basic principles of sound nutrition outlined in this book. Don't try for perfection, try for improvements.

Now take a deep breath, get ready, and start building your foundation!

Week 1: Laying The Foundation

Exercise	Date: Weight / Reps	Date: Weight / Reps	Date: Weight / Reps
Squat			
Straight-arm pullover			
Squat			
Straight-arm pullover			
Stiff-legged deadlift			
Bench press			
Behind-neck press			
Pull-up			
Parallel dip			
Abdominal crunches			

Week #:   **Date:**   **Daily Calories:**

<u>Breakfast</u>

Food Group	Food	Servings

Week #:   **Date:**   **Daily Calories:**

Morning snack		
Food Group	Food	Servings

Week #:   **Date:**   **Daily Calories:**

Lunch		
Food Group	Food	Servings

Week #:	Date:	Daily Calories:

Afternoon snack

Food Group	Food	Servings

Week #:   **Date:**   **Daily Calories:**

Dinner		
Food Group	Food	Servings

Week #:   **Date:**   **Daily Calories:**

Night time snack

Food Group	Food	Servings

Week 2: Laying The Foundation

Exercise	Date: Weight / Reps	Date: Weight / Reps	Date: Weight / Reps
Squat			
Straight-arm pullover			
Squat			
Straight-arm pullover			
Stiff-legged deadlift			
Bench press			
Behind-neck press			
Pull-up			
Parallel dip			
Abdominal crunches			

Week #:   **Date:**   **Daily Calories:**

Breakfast

Food Group	Food	Servings

Week #:   **Date:**   **Daily Calories:**

<u>Morning snack</u> Food Group	Food	Servings

Week #:   **Date:**   **Daily Calories:**

Lunch

Food Group	Food	Servings

Week #:	Date:	Daily Calories:
Afternoon snack		
Food Group	Food	Servings

Week #:   **Date:**   **Daily Calories:**

Dinner

Food Group	Food	Servings

Week #:	Date:	Daily Calories:
Night time snack		
Food Group	Food	Servings

Week 3: Laying The Foundation

Exercise	Date: Weight / Reps	Date: Weight / Reps	Date: Weight / Reps
Squat			
Straight-arm pullover			
Squat			
Straight-arm pullover			
Stiff-legged deadlift			
Bench press			
Behind-neck press			
Pull-up			
Parallel dip			
Abdominal crunches			

Week #:   **Date:**   **Daily Calories:**

<u>Breakfast</u>

Food Group	Food	Servings

Week #:	Date:	Daily Calories:
Morning snack		
Food Group	Food	Servings

Week #:   **Date:**   **Daily Calories:**

Lunch

Food Group	Food	Servings

Week #:   **Date:**   **Daily Calories:**

Afternoon Snack

Food Group	Food	Servings

Week #: **Date:** **Daily Calories:**

<u>**Dinner**</u>		
Food Group	Food	Servings

Week #:	Date:	Daily Calories:
Night time snack		
Food Group	Food	Servings

10 Leg Work: Week 4

Great pillars of stone

Some of the oldest structures in the world still standing - primarily Greek and Roman buildings - featured massive stone pillars as an intregal part of their design. They were built to support enormous weight and to provide integrity and strength for the rest of the structure.

If you wanted to build a large building with a similar old Greek design, common sense dictates that you would build pillars large and strong enough to support it. The larger the building, the larger the pillars would need to be.

The human body, for the most part, follows the same commonsense, structural principles; It simply won't allow you to build a massive, muscular, stone-solid upper body, without the structure to support it.

So, now that you've built a strong foundation, let's begin working on your own great pillars of stone; The muscles of the legs.

The muscles of the legs are some of the largest and strongest in the human body. While they can be divided into several sections, for simplicity, they are generally seperated into four areas; the gluteus maximus, or "glutes" (the butt), the quadriceps, or " quads" (front of thigh), the biceps femoris, commonly called the "hamstrings" (back of thigh) and the gastrocnemius, or "calves" (lower back of leg). Taking time to develop these areas can lead to real benefits in terms of health, functional strength and overall muscular development throughout your entire body;

This week we will be using a double pre-exhaustion routine concentrating on the muscles of the leg. As mentioned earlier, pre-exhaustion is a technique used to drive a muscle past the point of exhaustion by combining single-joint and multiple-joint exercises for the same muscle group back to back. (see chapter 2 for a more detailed explanation). This is a *double* pre-exhaustion routine, meaning there are two, seperate pre-exhaustion cycles.   Start the first cycle with a set of leg extensions. Use the weight you would normally use and work to the point of failure. Immediately following the point of failure, move over to the leg press machine. You will need to reduce the weight that you would normally use by about 30%. It is important that you remember to switch exercises in 3 seconds or less. Allowing more than 3 seconds between exercises will significantly reduce the effects of the pre-exhaustion cycle. Again, perform as many repetitions as you can in good form until failure.

After a short break, move on to the second pre-exhaustion cycle; Start out by performing a set of leg curls using the weight you would normally use. After reaching momentary muscular failure, immediately perform a set of full squats. The weight will have to be reduced by 30 - 40%. Perform as many repetitons as possible.   When you can no longer perform a repetition in good form, stop and move on to the calf raise. Perform as many repetitions as you can (which probably won't be very many).

That completes the pre-exhaustion leg cycle. After a short break, you'll round out the workout with a few basic movements for the rest of the body.

A few pre-exhaustion cycles like this and you'll be well on your way to building strong, muscular legs and, in turn, a strong, muscular upper body.

Week 4: Leg Work

Exercise	Date: Weight / Reps	Date: Weight / Reps	Date: Weight / Reps
Leg extension			
Leg press			
Leg curl			
Squat			
Calf raise			
Bench press			
Barbell row			
Behind- neck press			
Barbell curl			
Triceps extension			
Abdominal crunch			

Week #:   **Date:**   **Daily Calories:**

Breakfast		
Food Group	Food	Servings

Week #:   **Date:**   **Daily Calories:**

Morning snack		
Food Group	Food	Servings

Week #:   **Date:**   **Daily Calories:**

<u>Lunch</u>

Food Group	Food	Servings

Week #:	**Date:**	**Daily Calories:**
Afternoon snack		
Food Group	Food	Servings

Week #:   **Date:**   **Daily Calories:**

Dinner

Food Group	Food	Servings

Week #:   **Date:**   **Daily Calories:**

Night time snack		
Food Group	Food	Servings

11 Arm Designs: Week 5

Thick cables of steel

Some of the largest and most impressive bridges in the world are supported, in part, by gigantic, thick cables of steel. This allows the bridge to hold a great deal of weight. Much more so, obviously, than a bridge supported by a weaker material, such as wood or rope.

In a similar way, your upper arms serve to hold and support in a very real-life functional way. In fact, developing the muscles of the upper arms(biceps & triceps), is one of the best ways to improve functional strength, and is probably one of the improvements you will notice most in your daily life; When you think about how often the arms are used in day-to-day activities - carrying groceries, lifting the kids, taking out the garbage and so on - you can begin to imagine how strengthening these muscles could make life just a little bit easier.

Strengthening the arms into strong, solid cables of steel requires a little bit of work, however, so... let's begin...

This week you will be performing another pre-exhaustion routine. Start out with a set of pull-ups immediately followed by a set of preacher curls. Again, the same rules apply as last week: No more than three seconds rest between exercises, and reduce the weight on the second exercise (preacher curls)to 30% of what you would use normally. Next, move immediately to the lat pulldown. That completes your first pre-exhaustion cycle.

After a short break(5 minutes or so), start your second pre-exhaustion cycle with a set of bench presses. As always, work until failure with your usual amount of weight. Next, move onto the triceps extension, and finally, finish off with a set of parallel dips. If you find it difficult to perfom even 1 or 2 repetitions on the dip, try doing 3 or 4 negative reps by stepping up to the top position and lowering yourself slowly.

After a breif rest, finish out the routine with the following basic exercises; Squat, straight-arm pullover, barbell row, reverse shoulder shrug, abdominal crnches, and hyper-extensions. Use the weight you would normally use, and perform them in the regular manner, or, if you wish, try applying the progressive negative tension technique(see chapter 2).

At this point in your training you should be noticing quite a bit of new muscle(perhaps in places you didn't even know you had muscle!) and you should be significantly stronger on all your exercises. Take time to evaluate your progress; you may want to measure the difference between your relaxed and flexed bicep, or take some skinfold measurements at this point. You may also want to weigh yourself and take a few circumference measurements of your waist, upper arms, chest and thighs. If you find that your skinfold or waist measurments have increased, you may want to consider reducing your caloric intake slightly, or increasing your aerobic activity. Don't be too concerned about body weight, however. An increase in body weight does not necessarily mean an increase in fat. You are in the process of building lots of new muscle tissue, and remember - muscle weighs more than fat.

Whatever your progress, be proud of your achievements. Building a great body - like building a great bridge or cathedral - takes hard work, time and patience....

Week 5: Arm Designs

Exercise	Date: Weight / Reps	Date: Weight / Reps	Date: Weight / Reps
Pull-up			
Preacher curl			
Pulldown behind neck			
Bench press			
Tricep extension			
Parallel dip			
Squat			
Straight-arm pullover			
Barbell row			
Reverse shoulder shrug			
Abdominal crunch			
Hyper-extension			

Week #:   **Date:**   **Daily Calories:**

Breakfast
Food Group   Food   Servings

Week #:   **Date:**   **Daily Calories:**

Morning snack

Food Group	Food	Servings

Week #:   **Date:**   **Daily Calories:**

Lunch
Food Group	Food	Servings

Week #:   **Date:**   **Daily Calories:**

Afternoon snack		
Food Group	Food	Servings

Week #: **Date:** **Daily Calories:**

Dinner		
Food Group	Food	Servings

Week #:   **Date:**   **Daily Calories:**

Night time snack		
Food Group	Food	Servings

12 Chest Expansion: Week 6

Massive slabs of rock

America's Stonehenge, in Salem, NH, contains some of the the oldest man-made structures in the United States. Carbon dating has suggested that they were built somewhere between 2,000 to 2,500 b.c. The site consists of many massive slabs of thick rock, crudely honed and assembled into primitive walls, huts, tunnels and tables. Crude, perhaps, but certainly enduring and functional.

As you work on building your chest muscles this week, think about those massive slabs of stone. Our goal is to build something just as solid, enduring and functional.

In order to build your massive, solid chest, this week we will be using another double pre-exhaustion routine;

The first pre-exhaustion cycle will start off with a set decline bench press. Immediately following(3 seconds or less) you will perform a set of bent-arm flyes with about 30% less weight than you would normally use. Finish the cycle off with a set of parallel dips.

After a short rest, start on the second pre-exhaustion cycle. Begin with a set of standard bench presses, then move on, again, to the bent-arm flye. Immediately following the bent-arm fly, move over to parallel dips, and finally, finish of the cycle by performing some push-ups. It is unlikely that you will be able to do more than 2 or 3 push-ups, but try anyway.

That completes the double pre-exhaustion cycle for this week. Finish up the routine with some basic exercises and feel free to experiment with some other techniques, such as forced reps, negatives, etc.

Building massive slabs of muscle on your chest is not easy, but following the routine in this chapter will assure that you attain a bigger and better chest - one that will be strong, functional, enduring and impressive - just like those ancient carved rocks at America's Stonehenge.

Week 6: Chest Expansion

Exercise	Date: Weight / Reps	Date: Weight / Reps	Date: Weight / Reps
Decline bench press			
Bent-arm flye			
Parallel dip			
Bench press			
Bent-arm flye			
Parallel dip			
Push-up			
Stiff-legged deadlift			
Straight-arm pullover			
Preacher curl			
Tricep extension			

Week #:   **Date:**   **Daily Calories:**

Breakfast Food Group	Food	Servings

Week #:	Date:	Daily Calories:
Morning snack		
Food Group	Food	Servings

Week #:   **Date:**   **Daily Calories:**

<u>**Lunch**</u>

Food Group	Food	Servings

Week #:   **Date:**   **Daily Calories:**

Afternoon snack

Food Group	Food	Servings

Week #:   **Date:**   **Daily Calories:**

<u>Dinner</u>

Food Group	Food	Servings

Week #:	Date:	Daily Calories:
Night time snack		
Food Group	Food	Servings

13 Back Issues: Week 7

Giant pyramids of Egypt

Most would agree that Egypt's ancient pyramids are some of the most impressive structures in human history. These massive works of art inspire an aura of mystery and awe like few other structures can. Stretching like mammoth triangular mountains into the desert sky, these pyramids are truly a testament to human ambition and ingenuity.

Surprisingly, the pyramids look much the same as they did 4,500 years ago when they were first constructed. The builders designed them to last for thousands of years, and they succeeded.

It took smart planning, hard physical work , patience and dedication to build the pyramids, and it will take the same to build a huge, flaring v-shaped back.

So, let's start building your own testament to human ambition and ingenuity - an inverted pyramid of muscle that will inspire awe in all who lay eyes upon it.....

Once again, we will be utilizing pre-exhaustion techniques this week as we specialize on the muscles of the back. First, we will start off with pull-ups, immediately followed by the bent-arm pullover, and finishing up with the lat pulldown. That will complete your first pre-exhaustion cycle. Take a breif rest(5 minutes or so), then start on your second pre-exhaustion cycle; Start by performing a set of barbell rows, immediately followed by bent-arm pullover, and ending with a set of behind-neck presses.

That completes the pre-exhaustion portion of your workout this week. Finish out your routine by performing one set each of the following exercises: Stiff-legged deadlift, leg extension, leg curl, calve raises, shoulder shrug, abdominal crunches and hyperextensions.

Feel free to experiment with some of the specialized

techniques this week also.... and when you feel discouraged or ready to quit, think of those giant pyramids, and how hard work, patience and dedication helped to achieve a great and inspiring vision.

Week 7: Back Issues

Exercise	Date: Weight / Reps	Date: Weight / Reps	Date: Weight / Reps
Pull-up			
Bent-arm pullover			
Pulldown behind neck			
Barbell row			
Bent-arm pullover			
Behind-neck press			
Stiff-legged deadlift			
Leg extension			
Leg curl			
Calve raise			
Shoulder shrug			
Abdominal crunch			
Hyper-extension			

Week #:   **Date:**   **Daily Calories:**

| **Breakfast** | | |
Food Group	Food	Servings

Week #:	**Date:**	**Daily Calories:**
Morning snack		
Food Group	Food	Servings

Week #:   **Date:**   **Daily Calories:**

Lunch		
Food Group	Food	Servings

Week #:   **Date:**   **Daily Calories:**

<u>**Afternoon snack**</u>		
Food Group	Food	Servings

Week #:   **Date:**   **Daily Calories:**

<u>Dinner</u>
Food Group   Food   Servings

Week #:   **Date:**   **Daily Calories:**

Night time snack		
Food Group	Food	Servings

14 Shoulder Additions: Week 8

Mighty domes of marble

One of the most famous architectural wonders in the world is the Taj Mahal in India. The emperor of the time hired the best architects, engineers and craftsmen from all over the world to build this remarkable structure as a testament of his love for his late wife. Built almost entirely of white Italian marble, it is an awe-inspiring example of what can be accomplished when art, engineering and passion are successfully merged. One of it's most noticeable and impressive characteristics is it's perfect symmetry. Inside and out, everything is deliberately balanced, from it's rectangular pools of water to it's perfectly placed towers. At its center sits an enormous white dome, and placed on each side like mighty bulging shoulders, two smaller, but equally impressive marble domes.

This week, as we focus on building the muscle of the shoulders, think about the importance of symmetry in structures and in the development of the body; Developing the muscle of the shoulders helps bring a sense of symmetry to the whole body. A well carved pair of shoulders can help even out and balance an otherwise flawed physique. So, let's start building your own mighty domes of marble...

This is your final week of training in this program, and we will start it with - you guessed it - a double pre-exhaustion routine; First, remember to warm-up and stretch, then start out by performing a set of overhead presses in good form. Immediately after, perform a set of lateral raises and finally finish off with a set of behind neck presses. After a short break, start your next pre-exhaustion set; it consists of performing a set of behind neck presses, immediately followed by the bent over raise and ending up with a set of upright rows. Finish up your routine with the following basic exercises: Stiff legged deadlift, leg extension, leg curl, bent-arm flye, biceps curl and triceps extension.

Week 8: Shoulder Additions

Exercise	Date: Weight / Reps	Date: Weight / Reps	Date: Weight / Reps
Overhead press			
Lateral raise			
Behind-neck press			
Behind-neck press			
Bent-over raise			
Upright row			
Stiff-legged deadlift			
Bench press			
Leg extension			
Leg curl			
Barbell curl			
Tricep extension			

Week #:   **Date:**   **Daily Calories:**

<u>**Breakfast**</u>
Food Group   Food   Servings

Week #:   **Date:**   **Daily Calories:**

Morning snack		
Food Group	Food	Servings

Week #:   **Date:**   **Daily Calories:**

Lunch

Food Group	Food	Servings

Week #:	Date:	Daily Calories:

Afternoon snack

Food Group	Food	Servings

Week #: **Date:** **Daily Calories:**

Dinner

Food Group	Food	Servings

Week #:	Date:	Daily Calories:

<u>Night time snack</u>

Food Group	Food	Servings

15 Evaluation

Evaluate your new body

A thorough evaluation of your new body can help you determine how much progress you've made throughout the program. After several weeks of training, it is sometimes easy to forget the condition you were in when you started. People often tend to ignore small, gradual improvements made along the way. So, let's take a good, clear look at the improvements you've made:

Bodyweight

Remember, a number of factors can determine bodyweight; fat to muscle ratio, bone density, water retention. As suggested before, use it as a *very general* guide to the changes in your body. Record your weight in the chart provided at the end of this chapter(figure A), and compare it to the weight recorded in chapter 8.

Body measurements

All measurements should be taken "cold", that is, before working out, without a muscle "pump". The tape should be pulled tight *against* the skin, but not so tight that it presses *into* the skin. Measure the following areas and record them in the chart provided at the end of this chapter(figure B): Calves, thighs, hips, waist, chest, forearms, upper arms and neck. Refer to chapter 8 - Preliminaries -for details.

Bodyfat

After eight weeks of hard training and proper eating, you should notice a significant decrease in bodyfat. Take a tricep skinfold measurement and a measurement of the difference between your relaxed and flexed upper arm and record your results in figure C.   Refer to chapter eight for details on performing these tests and interpreting the corresponding bodyfat percentages. Compare your results with those from eight weeks ago.

Before and after photos

Often, it only becomes clear that dramatic improvements were made after examining the before and after photos. Measurements speak the truth, but, as the saying goes - seeing is believing. Repeat the poses you chose at the beginning of this program, and try to duplicate the conditions in which the photos were first taken; lighting, background, etc. Once you have the new photos, place them side by side with the old photos in the spaces provided. Be sure to look closely at the details and try to notice the changes in all areas - even the small ones.

Strength

At the start of this program you tested your strength and neurological efficiency for your upper and lower body. While neurological efficiency is unlikely to change, your strength should have increased significantly - 30% to 40% - over the course of eight weeks. Test your upper and lower body strength in the following manner:

For upper body:

1. Start by warming up with the biceps curl; choose a weight that will allow you to perform 10-15 repetitions in very strict form. Stop short of momentary muscular failure.

2. Rest 3-5 minutes.

3. On the biceps curl, choose a weight that will only allow

    you to perform 1 repetition in good form. This is inherently dangerous - so be careful to avoid jerking or "throwing" the weight around. Perform the repetition with strict, controlled movement, and stop immediately if you experience any pain.

For lower body:

1. Start by warming up on the leg extension; choose a

weight that will allow you to perform 10-15 repetitions in very strict form. Stop short of momentary muscular failure.

2. Rest 3-5 minutes.

3. On the leg extension, choose a weight that will only allow you to perform 1 repetition in good form. This is inherently dangerous - so be careful to avoid jerking or "throwing" the weight around. Perform the repetition with strict, controlled movement, and stop immediately if you experience any pain.

Bodyweight (figure A)

Before

Date:	Weight in pounds

After

Date:	Weight in pounds

Body measurements (figure B)
Circumference(in inches)

	Week 1	Week 8	Difference
Right Calve			
Left Calve			
Right Thigh			
Left Thigh			
Hips			
Waist			
Chest			
Right Forearm			
Left Forearm			
Right Upper Arm			
Left Upper Arm			
Neck			

Bodyfat measurement (figure C)

Before

Triceps skinfold (mm)	Bodyfat %

Relaxed bicep (mm)	Flexed bicep (mm)	Difference

After

Triceps skinfold (mm)	Bodyfat %

Relaxed bicep (mm)	Flexed bicep (mm)	Difference

Strength test (figure D)

Before

Biceps curl	Leg extension
Weight (1 repetition max.)	

After

Before & After Photographs

Front - relaxed

Before

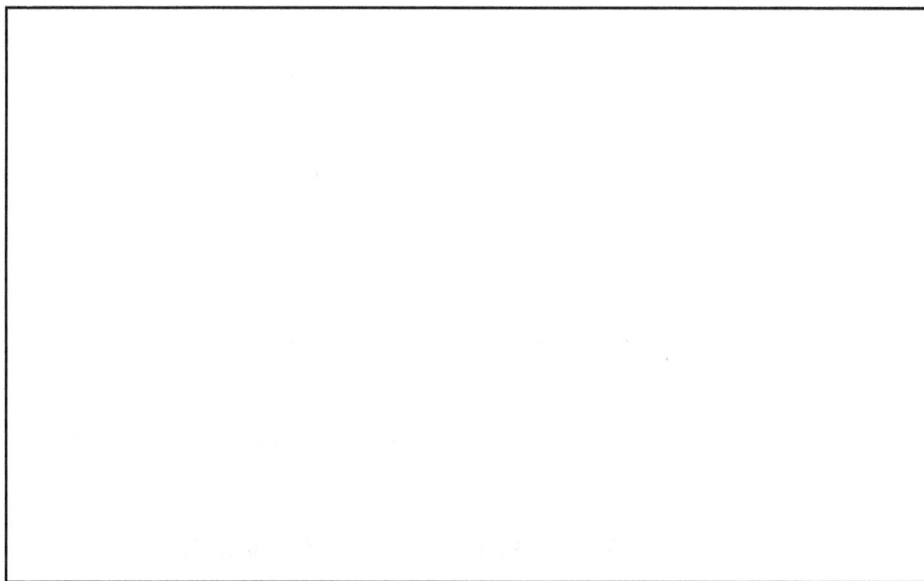

After

<u>Back - relaxed</u>

Before

After

<u>Right side - relaxed</u>

Before

After

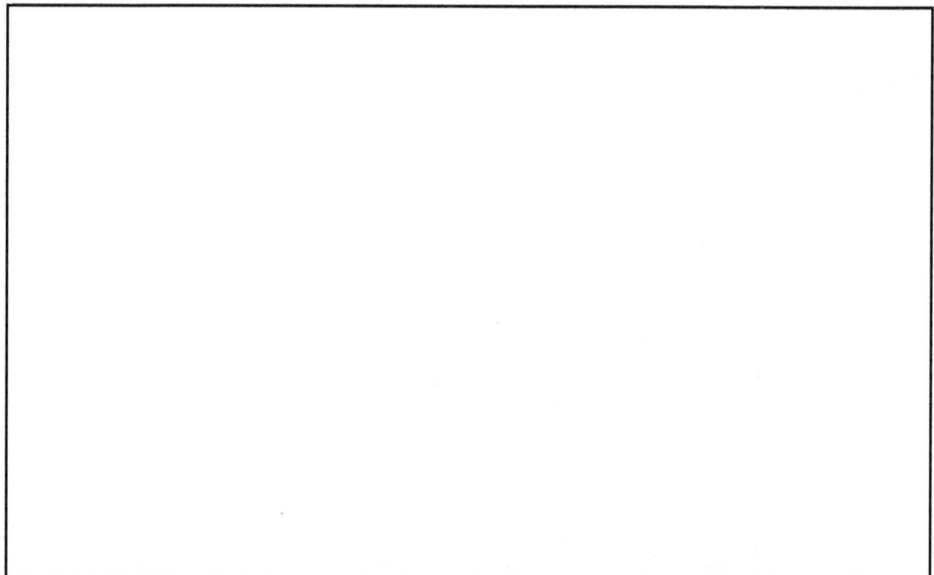

<u>Left side - relaxed</u>

Before

After

<u>Pose 1 - flexed</u>

Before

After

Pose 2 - flexed

Before

After

Where do I
go from here?

Now that you've completed eight weeks of hard training and done a thorough evaluation of your progress, you may want to consider taking a short break from your training; Taking four or fives days off can do wonders for your recuperation and can prepare you for more advanced routines later on. It will also provide you with a good chance to decide exactly what your next goals will be; Would you like to continue to develop strength and muscle size? Maybe you would like to lose more body fat and develp more definition. Or are you happy with the way you look and just want to maintain?

Asking yourself questions like these and setting specific goals will help you to decide what type of training routine you should pursue next. If you should decide to continue your pursuit of strength and muscle size, consider repeating this entire eight week program (after a four or five day break) before moving on to any advanced training. Doing so will ensure that you are strong and advanced enough to try more intense and challenging routines. Remember, concentration on the basics will result in great advances in overall muscle strength and size.

What ever direction you decide to take with your training, remember that your body truly is a temple. Building a strong, beautiful one takes smart planning, passion, dedication, hard work and patience... just as it does to build any great structure.... from the pyramids of Egypt to the Taj Mahal....

Index

V

W

Z

NOTES

For **FREE INFORMATION** on other health, fitness and self-improvement books and articles send name and address to:

**ANTHEM PRESS
POST OFFICE BOX 33
EAST DERRY, NH 03041**

Or, check us out online at: www.anthem-press.com

Also by Steven C. Cummings:

Increasing Height Through Exercise: Growth Theory & Practice

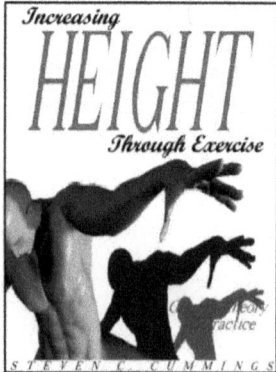

This is the original, best-selling classic that started the "height increase" and "grow taller" craze that swept the internet back in 1999/2000! Dozens, if not hundreds of imitators have since cropped up, all promising height increase, riches, the moon and everything else. But there is only one "Increasing Height Through Exercise", and it truly is the "bible" of height increase information. Don't settle for cheap imitations and knock-offs, go back to the source: The original "Increasing Height Through Exercise", circa, 2000. It's the grand-daddy of the "grow taller" industry and it will show you:

▸ Which exercises to perform for maximum possible height increase in minimum time.

▸ How to use simple, inexpensive devices to make you taller, faster.

▸ How to use common, easy to find supplements proven to build and repair cartilage for the best results from your exercise routine.

▸ How to gain permanent, fool-proof height increases (up to 6 inches!)using proven but radical new therapies, such as: artificial intervertebral disc implants, bone lengthening surgery and human growth hormone treatments.

▸ Mind-bending psychological techniques to enhance your growth results, including neuro-linguistic programming, hypnosis and lucid dreaming !

And there is much, much more...

To find out more about Increasing Height Through Exercise, or to order a copy, go to amazon.com or anthem-press.com

www.ingramcontent.com/pod-product-compliance
Lightning Source LLC
Chambersburg PA
CBHW080330270326
41927CB00014B/3166